About Island Press

Since 1984, the nonprofit organization Island Press has been stimulating, shaping, and communicating ideas that are essential for solving environmental problems worldwide. With more than 800 titles in print and some 40 new releases each year, we are the nation's leading publisher on environmental issues. We identify innovative thinkers and emerging trends in the environmental field. We work with world-renowned experts and authors to develop cross-disciplinary solutions to environmental challenges.

Island Press designs and executes educational campaigns in conjunction with our authors to communicate their critical messages in print, in person, and online using the latest technologies, innovative programs, and the media. Our goal is to reach targeted audiences—scientists, policymakers, environmental advocates, urban planners, the media, and concerned citizens—with information that can be used to create the framework for long-term ecological health and human well-being.

Island Press gratefully acknowledges major support of our work by The Agua Fund, The Andrew W. Mellon Foundation, Betsy & Jesse Fink Foundation, The Bobolink Foundation, The Curtis and Edith Munson Foundation, Forrest C. and Frances H. Lattner Foundation, G.O. Forward Fund of the Saint Paul Foundation, Gordon and Betty Moore Foundation, The Kresge Foundation, The Margaret A. Cargill Foundation, New Mexico Water Initiative, a project of Hanuman Foundation, The Overbrook Foundation, The S.D. Bechtel, Jr. Foundation, The Summit Charitable Foundation, Inc., V. Kann Rasmussen Foundation, The Wallace Alexander Gerbode Foundation, and other generous supporters.

The opinions expressed in this book are those of the author(s) and do not necessarily reflect the views of our supporters.

Whitewash

Whitewash

THE STORY OF A WEED KILLER, CANCER,
AND THE CORRUPTION OF SCIENCE

WITHDRAWN

Carey Gillam

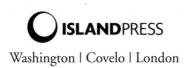

ISLANDPRESS

Washington | Covelo | London

Island Press would like to thank Deborah Wiley for generously supporting the publication of this book.

Library of Congress Control Number: 2017940669

All Island Press books are printed on environmentally responsible materials.

Manufactured in the United States of America
10 9 8 7 6 5 4 3 2

Keywords: agrichemicals, Environmental Protection Agency (EPA), genetically modified organisms (GMOs), glyphosate, herbicide, Monsanto, non-Hodgkin's lymphoma (NHL), pesticide resistance, Roundup, United States Department of Agriculture (USDA)

For the farmers who have given me their time, shared their wisdom, and helped me understand the obstacles they face as they work to feed us all.

Agriculture . . . is our wisest pursuit, because it will in the end contribute most to real wealth, good morals and happiness.

—Thomas Jefferson,
letter to George Washington, 1787

Contents

Preface   xi

Introduction: A Silent Stalker   1

Chapter 1. What Killed Jack McCall?   7

Chapter 2. An Award-Winning Discovery   23

Chapter 3. The "Roundup Ready" Rollout   43

Chapter 4. Weed Killer for Breakfast   55

Chapter 5. Under the Microscope   79

Chapter 6. Spinning the Science   113

Chapter 7. A Poisoned Paradise   135

Chapter 8. Angst in Argentina   153

Chapter 9. Uproar in Europe   169

Chapter 10. When Weeds Don't Die, But Butterflies Do   189

Chapter 11. Under the Influence   215

Chapter 12. Seeking Solutions   235

Epilogue   249

Acknowledgments   253

Notes   255

About the Author   295

Index   297

Preface

It's been nearly twenty years since I first walked into the corporate head-quarters of Monsanto Company, a visit that would become one of many over the course of my career as a national correspondent for Reuters, one of the oldest and largest news agencies in the world. Meeting with top executives, scientists, and marketing experts at Monsanto, perhaps the world's best-known agricultural powerhouse, was part of a job that called on me to help keep international audiences informed about the ins and outs and evolutions of agriculture in the United States. The types of seeds farmers plant in their fields and the chemicals they use to treat their crops are big business, amounting to billions of dollars in revenues for Monsanto and the other companies that sell them. But the fundamentals of growing food ultimately have much larger implications. Not only do farmers' choices influence commodity pricing and trade relationships, but they also ultimately affect the health and well-being of all of us. The food we eat, the water we drink, the landscape of our environment, all are connected to these seemingly simple choices made by farmers in their fields.

Before my 1998 move to the farm state of Kansas to write about agriculture for Reuters, I spent a good deal of my journalism career delving into the financial wheeling and dealing of the big banking, commercial real estate, and insurance industries. I also spent a fair share of my time chasing chaos—I covered the death and devastation wrought by Hurricane Katrina; floods, fires, and droughts; and the countless tornadoes that roared across rural America. And I was dispatched to duck bullets, bricks, and bottles in the race-torn riots of Ferguson, Missouri, and elsewhere.

When assigned to cover the "ag beat," I was at first a bit reluctant. I was skeptical that it could bring the intrigue and excitement I had experienced with the prior work I had done. And I had a lot to learn. My education in food production and farming meant not just sitting down with executives at companies such as Monsanto and its rivals Dow Agro-Sciences and DuPont but also listening to, and studying the work of, agricultural economists, soil and plant scientists, experts on seed germplasm, and—of course—farmers. My favorite times as an ag journalist have been spent in blue jeans and mud boots, traipsing through higher-than-my-head cornstalks with farmers and riding inside the cabs of combines alongside the hardworking, often tough-talking men and women who understand better than anyone the risks and rewards of modern food production. I have immense respect and gratitude for these farmers who devote their lives to toiling in unforgiving fields, where the harvest bounty often depends on the whims of Mother Nature and the bulk of the profits go to deep pockets much higher up the food chain. And I stand a bit in awe of the scientists who spend their careers studying how to do more with less, how to grow enough food for an expanding world population in ways that could not even have been imagined a generation ago.

When I started down that reporting road, I was an eager student, nearly as impressed with the advanced technologies of modern agriculture as with the people who work the land. I was someone who had never given much thought to what went into the products I purchased at the grocery store. I didn't buy organically grown produce, as it seemed too expensive, and I didn't spend time fretting over invisible chemicals that might lurk in my lunch. The debate about the then-nascent technique of making transgenic changes to food crops was a mystery to me. And I was a devoted consumer fan of Monsanto's hit herbicide product, Roundup, using it liberally in my suburban backyard to keep weeds at bay. Wide-eyed is the best way to describe my reaction to seeing Monsanto's "corn chipper" in action and to those initial visits to biotechnology crop demonstration fields. I became a fan of the company's chief technology officer, an engagingly brilliant, bald-headed scientist named Robb Fraley, and I always enjoyed my many chats with the affable Brett Begemann, who grew up on a Missouri grain and livestock farm before rising through the ranks to eventually become Monsanto's president.

But over the years, as my research and reporting expanded to include doubts about the benefits of genetically modified organisms and the risks associated with the chemicals used on them, I became a target of Monsanto's ire. Company representatives and industry surrogates alternately sought to bully me, charm me, intimidate me, and cajole me to write news stories in ways that parroted industry talking points. They told me there was no justification for reporting both sides of the debates over Monsanto's crops and chemicals because the science was settled, all was well, and anyone who questioned that was thwarting Monsanto's mission to "feed the world." When I would not adopt the desired narrative, surrogates attempted to assault my character and credibility and made efforts to derail my career. Monsanto executives and representatives from Monsanto-funded organizations sought unsuccessfully to convince my editors to yank me off my beat, to block further coverage of the issues. They could rarely, if ever, find errors in my reporting. The problem, they would complain, was one of "bias."

As you'll see in reading this book, the only bias I hold is for the truth. What I've learned, what I know with certainty, is that when powerful corporations control the narrative, the truth often gets lost, and it's up to journalists to find it and bring it home. That's what I've tried to do with this book. For decades, companies have whitewashed many of the facts about the crops and chemicals that they have helped make a central part of modern agriculture. Yes, there are rewards, but there are also risks—many. And without transparency, none of us can make informed decisions about what we eat and what policies we do or do not want to support.

My admiration for American farmers has never waned. But this journey through our nation's food system has left me with a very real fear—for my children, for your children—over what the future holds. It is undeniable that we've allowed our food, our water, our soil, our very selves to become dangerously doused with chemicals, and one of the most pervasive of those pesticides is the subject of this book.

Scientists call it glyphosate. Consumers know it as Roundup. It's a weed killer, but it's killing much more than weeds. And the regulatory agencies charged with protecting the public from these dangers have acted—intentionally or not—in ways that have protected corporate products and profits instead of people. It's not a feel-good story. But it is one that has to be told.

A Silent Stalker

If we are going to live so intimately with these chemicals—eating and drinking them, taking them into the very marrow of our bones—we had better know something about their nature and their power.

—Rachel Carson, *Silent Spring*

Since the mid-1990s, one of the largest and loudest public policy debates in the United States and Europe has been over the introduction of genetically engineered crops. Questions about the safety of these crops—for humans, animals, and the environment—have raged across continents, roiling markets and dividing nations and states over how to view this type of tinkering with nature. The debate has led to increasing consumer awareness of, and activism against, the industrialized farming practices that produce our food, and numerous books have documented an array of concerns over genetically modified crops.

But shadowing the controversy over genetically modified organisms (GMOs) is what I believe to be the *true* health and environmental calamity of modern-day biotech agriculture—the flood across our landscape of the pesticide known by chemists as glyphosate and by the rest of us simply as Roundup. From the day genetically engineered crops were introduced, they were designed with one primary purpose in mind—to withstand treatments of glyphosate, the highly efficient and effective weed-killing ingredient in Monsanto Company's Roundup branded herbicides. Farmers using Monsanto's Roundup Ready seeds along with Roundup herbicide could knock weeds out of their fields without worrying about killing their crops. Then and now, most of the genetically modified crops grown in the world carry the glyphosate-tolerant trait, enabling and encouraging farmers to choose to use this herbicide over any other on their farm fields. It was a brilliant move by Monsanto and made the company billions of dollars in combined sales of seeds and herbicide. But it has cost the rest of us, and generations yet to come, in ways impossible to calculate.

Just as dichlorodiphenyltrichloroethane, or DDT—now banned because of environmental and health risks—once was widely used as an insecticide the world over and declared "a benefactor of all humanity,"[1] glyphosate was heralded as a "one in a 100-year discovery that is as important for reliable global food production as penicillin is for battling disease."[2]

And just as the truth of DDT's dangers eventually came to light, the devastation wrought by years of nearly unchecked use of Roundup and other glyphosate-based weed killers has emerged as another example of how influential corporate interests can trump protection of the public.

The story of how this once obscure chemical became a common household name shows that the lessons of Rachel Carson and her book *Silent Spring* appear to have been forgotten as man-made dependence on glyphosate and other synthetic pesticides wreaks havoc on people, animals, and the land. As before, it begins with power, money, and politics, which have combined to accelerate glyphosate's use to unprecedented levels and have inserted this toxic pesticide into the diets of people around the world. Many have suffered deadly diseases linked to glyphosate, while scientists who raise red flags about these risks have been bullied and ostracized. Their experiences are recorded in these pages, as are efforts by regulators to straddle the fence between protecting public health and appeasing moneyed interests. Internal documents and communications, obtained through Freedom of Information Act (FOIA) requests, make clear how corporate players and a consortium of public and private scientists have manipulated regulators and lawmakers into green-lighting ever-higher uses of this chemical even as danger signs mounted.

Amid the growing crisis, consumers are awakening to the fact that they must hold regulators and lawmakers accountable for the levels of glyphosate and other pesticides in the foods we all eat. Concerns about glyphosate residues were part of the push for GMO labeling, and they drove consumer and environmental groups to petition regulators in the European Union and the United States to block further use of the chemical in 2016. European Parliament members took the concerns so seriously that in early 2016 they had their urine tested for glyphosate—finding alarming results—and some U.S. moms and researchers started testing breast milk and an array of foods. Fears about glyphosate also have started to affect international trade. Oatmeal products from the United States were rejected in the spring of 2016 by food inspectors in Taiwan because they contained glyphosate traces. Glyphosate is such a hot topic that industry players established a Twitter feed for the pesticide in March 2015.

Use of glyphosate has skyrocketed in the past twenty years, in part because as Monsanto's patent on the chemical was nearing expiration in the year 2000, the company introduced glyphosate-tolerant soybeans, corn, canola, sugar beets, and other crops, linking its new crop technology to its older chemical agent. Genetically engineered alfalfa, a common food for livestock, is also regularly doused with glyphosate now. Monsanto also encouraged farmers to use glyphosate—not on top of crops but as a traditional herbicide—in the production of hundreds of other foods that are not genetically engineered, including wheat, oats, vegetables, fruits, and nuts. U.S. farmers alone applied about 276 million pounds in 2014, compared with 40 million pounds in 1995, according to published research, and use globally has more than doubled in just the past ten years.[3] Around the globe, glyphosate is now registered for use in 130 countries and is manufactured by dozens of producers following Monsanto's lead. It is considered the most heavily used agricultural chemical in history.[4]

The popularity of glyphosate has been a boon for companies using it in their herbicide products. But emerging research in recent years is showing a host of unforeseen problems for people and the environment, including evidence that glyphosate may be a human carcinogen and that residues of this potentially cancer-causing chemical are frequently found in an array of popular foods, including cereals and snacks. Heavy use of glyphosate has also been showing detrimental effects on soil biology, which in turn affects the health and nutritional profile of crops. And use of the chemical has spawned what scientists and farmers have nicknamed "superweeds"—weeds that can grow several feet tall, choking off important food crops, and that are largely impervious to efforts to wipe them out. These superweeds now cost U.S. farmers billions of dollars per year in added labor and chemicals and lost production. The evidence is still evolving but already makes it clear that this weed killer, which for decades was believed to be benign—"safe enough to drink," according to some promoters—is endangering public and environmental health much more than the altered DNA of the crops it is tied to. It is not the most inherently dangerous of pesticides on the market, but its broad use for everything from farm fields to golf courses gives it a reach into every avenue of our lives, far deeper than that of other agrochemicals.

Indeed, recent government and academic research shows that glyphosate is pervasive in water, in air, and in our food. Just how much of the pesticide we've been consuming has been hard to determine, thanks largely to a U.S. regulatory community that has repeatedly said there is no need to test for glyphosate because the agrochemical industry has proven it to be so safe. In fact, glyphosate stands out as the one widely used pesticide that has not been included in years of annual government surveys of pesticide residues in food. Both the U.S. Food and Drug Administration (FDA) and the U.S. Department of Agriculture (USDA) annually test thousands of food products for hundreds of different types of pesticide residues, but both routinely have refused to test for glyphosate.

It's also notable that as the USDA and FDA have been declining to test for glyphosate residues over the past twenty years, the U.S. Environmental Protection Agency (EPA), which regulates pesticides, has been approving industry requests for higher and higher allowable levels of glyphosate residues in food. In 2013, for example, the EPA, at the request of Monsanto, raised the legally allowed amount of glyphosate residues in food considered safe to levels far higher than in other countries.

Disquiet about the safety of this widely used pesticide is global. Scientists and academics around the world have been trying to sound an alarm for years as growing use of glyphosate has tracked with mounting evidence of its dangers. The scientists warn that animal and epidemiology studies published in the past decade raise serious concerns about glyphosate's safety. There are strong indications that the chemical could trigger endocrine disruption, hormone system disturbances that have been linked to some cancers, birth defects, and developmental problems in children.

This book takes readers deep into the data and reveals not only how corporations keep a tight rein on regulators but also how they push "science" that supports their profit-focused interests to the forefront— all while burying evidence of harm. Documents obtained from inside government agencies and state university research programs provide numerous examples of how the agrochemical industry has secretly funded "independent" professors and other scientists to lobby on behalf of glyphosate's safety; how the industry has quietly set up front groups and think tanks to support its interests; and how it has attacked and tried to discredit scientists who have spoken out. Its reach even extends into the USDA and EPA and the suppression of scientific findings by government agricultural researchers.

This particular pesticide—glyphosate—is only one of scores of chemicals that have taken root in our lives, offering profits for the corporations that sell them but perils for people exposed to them. Indeed, there is a large and expanding body of evidence tying various pesticide exposures to elevated rates of chronic diseases, including a range of cancers, diabetes, neurodegenerative disorders such as Parkinson's disease and Alzheimer's disease, birth defects, and reproductive disorders.

But the story of the world's most widely used weed killer illustrates how destructive the consequences can be when we allow the balancing of risk and reward to tip too far in the direction of danger.

CHAPTER 1

What Killed Jack McCall?

Standing on the ridge overlooking her coastal California farm, Teri McCall sees her late husband, Jack, nearly everywhere. There, atop the highest hill, is where the couple married in 1975—two self-described "hippies" who knew more about how to surf than to farm. Midway up the hill, on a lush plateau surrounded by the lemon, avocado, and orange trees Jack planted, sits the 800-square-foot house the then-young Vietnam War veteran built for his bride and a family that grew to include two sons and a daughter. One of those sons now lives there with his own wife and small son. Solar panels Jack set up in a sun-drenched stretch of grass help power the farm's irrigation system.

Down there, nestled in a velvety green valley, is the century-old farmhouse Jack and Teri made their home after Jack's parents died. The two-story white Victorian boasts a front porch wide enough for rocking chairs and potted flowers and for friends to gather. Jack and Teri spent countless quiet nights on that porch, watching stars light up the sky, which is always so dark out here in the countryside. Over the front door is a stained-glass window Jack installed that features a heart and flowers. Inside, a plaque etched with the word "Blessed" hangs over the bedroom door.

Teri was only seventeen when she met twenty-three-year-old Jack just after he returned from Vietnam. He had been a first lieutenant in the 101st Airborne Division and received both a Bronze Star and a Distinguished Flying Cross for his service. When Teri saw him, though, he didn't look like a soldier but more like a big kid, laughing and playing Frisbee with friends. She remembers being almost instantly smitten by his rugged good looks and easy smile. It took five years before they became more than friends, and then forty years passed all too quickly.

"Literally hundreds of times a day, something reminds me of him," McCall tells me as I stand beside her on the ridge one bright spring morning a few months after Jack's death. Her tears start to flow. "That's part of why it's so hard to believe . . . to know that even if I search the whole world, look everywhere, I can't find him now." She shakes her head. "So hard to believe I can never see him again."[1]

~

Anthony "Jack" McCall, age sixty-nine, died on December 26, 2015, after a painful and perplexing battle with an aggressive form of non-Hodgkin lymphoma, a type of cancer that forms in the lymphatic system and can appear almost anywhere in the body. The loss is certain, fixed forever in his family's heartbreak. But questions about why and how he was stricken—a man who never smoked, who stayed fit, and who had no history of cancer in his family—swirl around his use of the popular weed killer Roundup and its active ingredient, glyphosate.

McCall shunned pesticide use on his farm, except for Roundup. He didn't like the idea of synthetic chemicals floating around the orchard, where he grew apricots, peaches, plums, and apples, or near his precious avocados. But Roundup was marketed as having extremely low toxicity, nothing that a small farmer like Jack needed to worry about. He would drive twenty to thirty miles from his farm, just outside the seaside village of Cambria, to Morro Bay, or often into San Luis Obispo, to buy his favorite weed killer. He would then apply it himself, spraying the pesticide all around the farm to beat back worrisome weeds. He even recommended Roundup to friends in the small Cambria community, telling them it was supposed to be much safer than alternatives and touting its effectiveness.

In fact, this chemical called glyphosate has for many years been the most widely used herbicide in the world, in part because ever since its introduction in 1974 it has been marketed as one of the safest of all pesticides ever brought to market. Its developer, Monsanto Company, and other companies that started selling glyphosate-based herbicides after Monsanto's patent expired have collected billions of dollars in global sales off the well-known consumer and agricultural mainstay for eradicating troublesome weeds. Declared to be as safe as table salt, Roundup and other glyphosate products became the remedy of choice for millions of consumers, farmers, gardeners, and groundskeepers around the globe. It has been a preferred choice for use in city parks and on school playgrounds and to keep golf courses weed free. Monsanto has also promoted its weed killer for use in zoos.

But the death of McCall, and the illnesses and deaths of other farmers and glyphosate users like him, have come amid revelations of a number of hidden dangers associated with the chemical, including links to non-Hodgkin lymphoma. And what began as a trickle of worry has widened into a flood of outrage against Monsanto and the regulators who have deemed glyphosate safe. Soon after her husband's death, McCall's widow, Teri, joined a movement of thousands of people who are bringing wrongful death lawsuits against Monsanto—people from around the United States who claim that Roundup can cause cancer and that Monsanto has tried to cover up the risks.

As the fortieth anniversary of glyphosate's introduction to the market was notched in 2014, protests over its use mounted, not just in

America but also abroad. By early 2016, protesters in the United States, Europe, South America, and elsewhere were calling on regulators to restrict or ban glyphosate, citing scientific research linking it to a range of health and environmental ills. Regulators and private organizations started analyzing food, water, air, and soil for glyphosate residues, and fears about use of glyphosate on genetically engineered crops gave added ammunition to a grassroots groundswell calling for required labeling of foods containing genetically modified organisms (GMOs).

The evidence of glyphosate's dangers began building soon after the herbicide was introduced, but it wasn't until Monsanto's commercialization of genetically engineered crops designed to be sprayed directly with glyphosate—so-called Roundup Ready crops—that glyphosate use took off and, with it, signs of trouble.

The lawsuits began after a team of World Health Organization (WHO) cancer experts announced, in March 2015, that they had determined glyphosate was a probable human carcinogen. That team, from WHO's International Agency for Research on Cancer (IARC), said a review of many scientific studies showed that glyphosate had a positive association with non-Hodgkin lymphoma (NHL). This association was noteworthy because incidences of NHL had spiked over the past several decades, making it the tenth most common cancer worldwide, with nearly 386,000 new cases diagnosed in 2012. The statistics are especially concerning for those living in North America, where incidence rates are highest.[2]

Many scientists have been studying the rise in NHL seen over the past forty years, especially for farmworkers exposed to pesticides. And many have warned that glyphosate and Roundup could be contributing to a range of diseases and ailments. IARC's work did not constitute solid proof that glyphosate causes NHL or other health problems, of course, but it did offer authoritative analysis of research examining correlations between the pesticide and disease. The IARC team said their conclusions were based on "sufficient evidence of carcinogenicity" in studies of lab animals, "limited evidence" in humans, and evidence that glyphosate "caused DNA and chromosomal damage in human cells."[3]

"We should all minimize our use as much as possible," said Professor Lin Fritschi, an epidemiologist affiliated with Curtin University in Australia who specializes in studying occupational causes of cancer. Fritschi was part of the IARC team that evaluated glyphosate. "The people most at risk are people who use glyphosate a lot, such as farmers and gardeners, and they are the ones who should try and reduce their use," she said.[4]

In February 2016, Teri McCall became one of many people to act upon those warnings by taking their claims of glyphosate-related illnesses and deaths to court. Though Jack's death certificate blamed metastatic large cell lymphoma for his passing, his family believes the actual culprit was the chemical.

"Roundup was supposed to be safe," Teri's lawsuit states. "The truth, however, is far more insidious. The active chemical in Roundup, glyphosate, is a carcinogen, and Monsanto has known this fact for decades."[5]

Legal observers believe that the roughly 1,000 cancer claims filed between 2015 and early 2017 mark what is to become a mountain of legal actions targeting Monsanto and Roundup. Plaintiffs in several of the lawsuits make the same allegation, that Monsanto spent decades covering up signs of harm associated with the weed killer, even promoting falsified data. Monsanto "knew or should have known . . . that exposure to Roundup and specifically, its active ingredient glyphosate, could result in cancer and other severe illnesses and injuries," plaintiffs claim.[6] Monsanto has denied the allegations.

Many of the cases were centralized in federal court in San Francisco, to be handled by one judge in what promises to be a long and winding battle that could take years to litigate. Monsanto says that it empathizes with anyone facing cancer but insists there is no reliable scientific evidence showing that exposure to glyphosate or Roundup branded products can cause cancer. But the team of lawyers representing the plaintiffs say that Monsanto knowingly failed to warn customers about many dangers Roundup posed for human health. The lawyers—and several scientists—contend that Roundup is more dangerous than glyphosate alone because of an added ingredient that Monsanto used for many years to help the glyphosate adhere to plants. Some research has shown that this added ingredient, polyethoxylated tallow amine (POEA), can be extremely damaging to human cells. Regulators did not require extensive safety tests on the combination of glyphosate and POEA, and Monsanto did little such testing, plaintiffs allege. But this "secret soup," the plaintiffs claim, can be deadly.

Internal e-mails and other documents obtained by the plaintiffs' attorneys during the first rounds of court-ordered discovery show how hard Monsanto has worked over the years to defend itself against safety concerns associated with Roundup. In some e-mails, company executives discussed ghostwriting favorable research manuscripts that would appear to be authored by acclaimed independent scientists. In others, executives discussed recruiting and paying experts who would lend credibility to Monsanto's claims of product safety; and in one, a Monsanto executive stated how "useful" a certain senior official of the U.S. Environmental Protection Agency (EPA) could be in "glyphosate defense."[7] Court records show that same official went to work for Monsanto-related organizations almost immediately after retiring from the EPA. Taken together, the documents paint an alarming picture indicating that year after year, at crossroads after crossroads, when research raised concerns about glyphosate, Monsanto's response was to turn away from the warnings and work harder to promote more use of the chemical. EPA documents show that Monsanto even protested the worker safety rules the agency said needed to accompany glyphosate products, calling such cautionary requirements "unjustified."[8] The company also resisted recommendations from an EPA toxicologist that the word "Danger" be used instead of "Warning" on Roundup labels.[9]

Monsanto has argued that its internal communications taken individually do not accurately reflect the company's actions or intentions, and company attorneys tried to keep the documents sealed. But the federal judge overseeing the multidistrict litigation ruled that many could be made part of the public court file.

Mother, grandmother, and former coffee farmer Christine Sheppard hopes she lives long enough to see the outcome of her lawsuit against the company. Though her NHL was in remission when we last spoke, Sheppard's life changed irreparably when she was stricken with a vicious version of the cancer, which would steal not only her health but also the idyllic retirement she and her husband, Kenneth, had carved out for themselves on a coffee plantation in Hawaii. She was a healthy and happy forty-seven-year-old working as director of marketing for a software company, and her husband, slightly older, was an engineering manager at a hardware company, when the two decided they'd had enough of the fast pace of the high-tech industry and they'd try their hand at farming. The couple left their home in San Diego, California, and plowed their hefty savings into a five-acre former coffee farm on the Big Island of Hawaii, in the Kona coffee-growing region. They moved to the farm in 1996.

"The weeds were so high that we could hardly wade through them, and the coffee was trees instead of bushes, tall with many branches twisted together," Sheppard recalled.[10] To tackle the weeds, the Sheppards strapped on backpack herbicide applicators and walked through the groves, spraying Roundup generously. They repeated this routine at different points throughout the years to keep weeds at bay.

"We were just carrying on the practices that were common in the area," she said. "Roundup was standard for the coffee-growing region and was recommended by the University of Hawaii's agricultural agent there. The department of agriculture would put on conferences on how to spray it so it didn't hurt the coffee trees. We were told it was safe enough to drink and we didn't need to wear protective gear."

For many years, the Sheppards felt they were living their dream. They learned the coffee business quickly, built a website to market their fresh-roasted beans online, and sold the coffee to visitors who toured their farm. Sheppard became so involved that she was elected president of the area's Kona Coffee Council, and her husband acted as director of education, organizing seminars and workshops for other farmers. The farm also came to be an animal sanctuary of sorts as the couple brought home a menagerie of dogs, cats, donkeys, and goats. "Our life on the farm was wonderful," Sheppard recalled.

They were making a plan to transition their coffee to organic, purely as a marketing move, according to Sheppard, when her health took a sudden and worrisome turn. One leg swelled and throbbed, she was frequently fatigued, and she began having night sweats. At first she thought her symptoms marked the onset of menopause; then she thought she might have blood poisoning. A doctor prescribed blood thinners, to no avail. Subsequent tests revealed the startling diagnosis: Sheppard had stage 4 large B-cell non-Hodgkin lymphoma, with roughly a 10 percent chance of survival.

It was August 2003, and she immediately started on months of chemotherapy. By the summer of 2004, the couple had sold the farm, which they could no longer manage, and moved back to California for expensive and exhausting experimental treatments. The treatments ultimately were successful enough to move Sheppard into remission in 2005. She's been left with lasting neuropathy, which causes severe foot and hand pain; loss of balance; and a host of other ailments that make it difficult for her to get through a day without medications. And the couple's savings have been exhausted on medical bills. For years, Sheppard said, she would "beat on the walls and wonder 'why me?'"—until the spring of 2015, when she read about Roundup's ties to non-Hodgkin lymphoma.

"My anger is still pretty raw," Sheppard told me. "The way Monsanto is reacting, their efforts to discredit things, are typical of what the tobacco industry did when information was coming out about links to lung cancer. I know they're going to fight hard. And they've got deep pockets."

Monsanto faces a long list of people who attribute their cancers to Roundup. Texan Joselin Barrera, a daughter of migrant farmworkers, believes growing up in an environment where the pesticide was regularly sprayed gave her non-Hodgkin lymphoma. Elias de la Garza, a former migrant farmworker and landscaper, also from Texas, similarly claimed his NHL was due to Roundup exposure. Judi Fitzgerald, a horticultural worker diagnosed with leukemia in 2012, also filed suit. California sod farm worker Brenda Huerta, who was diagnosed with NHL in 2013, also sued Monsanto for allegedly hiding the dangers of glyphosate.

John Sanders worked for thirty years managing weeds in orange and grapefruit groves in Redlands, California, before he developed NHL. Frank Tanner owned a landscaping business in California and started using Roundup in 1974; he was diagnosed with NHL after years of spraying glyphosate. Both are suing.

Orange County, California, resident Goldie Perkins sued Monsanto in July 2016, claiming the non-Hodgkin lymphoma she was diagnosed with in July 2014 was caused by exposure to Roundup products that she started using in the 1970s. Perkins echoed others in her assertion that scientific fraud helped get and keep glyphosate products on the market for decades.

From all over the country, from small towns to large cities, people are alleging connections between disease and glyphosate-based Roundup and say they were intentionally led to trust in the safety of a product that was not truly safe. "Monsanto assured the public that Roundup was harmless. In order to prove this, Monsanto championed falsified data and attacked legitimate studies that revealed its dangers," states one lawsuit, filed by Enrique Rubio, who claims he got cancer after nearly twenty years of regular exposure to Roundup while working in strawberry and vegetable fields in Oregon, California, and Texas. "Monsanto led a prolonged campaign of misinformation to convince government agencies, farmers, and the general population that Roundup was safe," his lawsuit states.[11]

Monsanto fought to have the cases thrown out, but as of this writing they are moving forward, and legal experts warn that glyphosate-related liability litigation could persist for decades. Lawyers working on the cases say they believe they will prove that Monsanto has deliberately concealed information about the dangers of its herbicide, an implication that, if proven, could reverberate around the world, given the global pervasiveness of the chemical. The lawyers and many observers familiar with glyphosate's history expect the litigation to rival mass tort actions seen over harms associated with dichlorodiphenyltrichloroethane (DDT), asbestos, and polychlorinated biphenyls (PCBs).

Monsanto argues that forty years of studies show glyphosate to be extremely safe and not cancer-causing. The company has asserted that IARC's findings were based on "junk science" and that politically motivated scientists have unfairly maligned the chemical.[12] Monsanto hired its own team of experts in 2015 to review the safety of glyphosate and said they found no cancer links.

But IARC was not the first to link glyphosate to cancer. The EPA's own scientists had the very same concerns back in the mid-1980s. A 1985 internal memo details how agency scientists themselves classified glyphosate as a possible human carcinogen. It was six years later, after extensive input from Monsanto, that the agency switched its tune and declared instead that it found "evidence of non-carcinogenicity for humans."[13] The change was made over the objections of some peer review members involved in the classification.

By the mid-1990s, Monsanto was facing accusations about Round-up's safety by New York's attorney general, Dennis Vacco, who grew up working on his family's 3,000-acre farm raising snap beans and Concord grapes. Vacco sued Monsanto for allegedly using "false and misleading advertising," including assurances that Roundup could safely be used in areas where children and pets play.[14] The attorney general also challenged Monsanto for using phrases like "You can feel good" about using its glyphosate-based herbicides because they were "practically non-toxic." Monsanto did not admit wrongdoing but agreed to pay $50,000 and to stop making such advertising claims in New York. Advertising in other states was not affected.

Aaron Johnson, a farmworker from Hawaii who was diagnosed with non-Hodgkin lymphoma in 2014, said he relied on those claims of safety during the roughly twenty years that he spent living and working amid the pineapple, macadamia, and papaya farms of Pahoa, Hawaii. "They would say it was safe as table salt. That was a common belief," recalled Johnson, who is one of the plaintiffs in the Roundup litigation. He loved his life on the island, surfing and hiking and taking a morning jog through the fields before work each morning. When the sickness set in, Johnson said, he was blindsided by the news that he had blood cancer. He initially was told he had but three months to live. Johnson spent the next year undergoing chemotherapy and bone marrow transplant treatment before being declared by doctors to be in remission in 2015. He now tends to a small orchard of his own, hand-weeding and shunning any chemical herbicides, especially Roundup.

"I think that they've known since the '70s this stuff can cause cancer. And now, on the scale that it has been distributed and used . . . this molecule is everywhere, in our food, our water," Johnson said. "They say it can be found in every person. As time goes on we're going to find out that it is a lot bigger than people can even imagine right now. All for profit—all for the sake of making billions a year off this one product. I don't understand how they've been able to get away with it."[15]

Legal experts say it will take much more than heartrending stories to demonstrate that Monsanto bears responsibility for the disease that tore apart so many lives. Proving that Roundup caused an individual's cancer, and that the company knew of and covered up evidence of carcinogenicity, is a big legal hill to climb. Monsanto claims the best science proves the safety of its herbicide and argues that regulators around the world are on its side. With more than $15 billion in revenues in 2015 and a long track record of victories in court battles over other complaints about its practices and products, Monsanto has been undeterred by the mountain of lawsuits. Its arsenal to combat adversaries will become even stronger if a planned merger between Monsanto and Germany's Bayer AG is completed.

Still, the dozens of attorneys pushing the cases forward say they have strong evidence that Roundup is just the latest example of a pattern by Monsanto of making false safety claims and covering up evidence about a dangerous substance. Indeed, the Roundup litigation closely mirrors courtroom battles Monsanto fought for years involving the polychlorinated biphenyls, or PCBs, it once manufactured.

Plaintiffs in those cases claimed PCB exposure caused them to fall ill while Monsanto hid the risks. Monsanto claimed, as it has done in the Roundup cases, that plaintiffs could not definitively link illnesses to PCB exposure. But the court-ordered discovery process required Monsanto to turn over internal documents that demonstrated the company was aware of health and environmental hazards even as it worked to keep the public in the dark and manipulated scientific studies to downplay the risks of PCB exposure.

A St. Louis, Missouri, jury in May 2016 ordered Monsanto and affiliates to pay $46 million in the cases of three people from Alaska, Michigan, and Oklahoma who said that exposure to PCBs gave them or their loved ones non-Hodgkin lymphoma. As with glyphosate, Monsanto was the primary U.S. maker of PCBs, until Congress outlawed them in 1979. And like glyphosate, PCBs were once used prolifically, for everything from industrial equipment to food product packaging. Hundreds of other PCB cases have been tried or are progressing through courts. Monsanto still faces legal claims by state officials in Washington who allege the company's production of PCBs contaminated more than 600 sites around the state, polluting waterways as well as soil and air. The state contends Monsanto hid its knowledge of the dangers of PCBs for years.

In 2003, Monsanto and a company it spun off called Solutia, along with a company called Pharmacia, through which Monsanto operated briefly as a subsidiary, agreed to pay roughly $700 million to address claims by more than 20,000 plaintiffs over PCB contamination in Anniston, Alabama, where the company operated a PCB manufacturing plant.[16] Studies linked PCBs to diabetes and liver disease in the Anniston area, though Monsanto had said for years that PCBs were not endangering public health.[17]

Some scientists and environmental activists who have long followed the trails of chemical pollution believe the evolution of glyphosate also mirrors that of DDT, a common pesticide most famous for its ability to wipe out malaria-carrying mosquitoes. DDT was also used in agriculture and in residential areas, and, like glyphosate, it was viewed for decades as a near-magical chemical before it fell from favor amid evidence of dire health and environmental consequences. DDT was award winning—the 1948 Nobel Prize in Physiology or Medicine went to Swiss chemist Paul Hermann Müller, who discovered its insecticidal properties in 1939. The dangers of DDT took years to fully emerge, although—like glyphosate—DDT raised early red flags with scientists. After decades of use, DDT was found to be an endocrine disruptor, and, like glyphosate, it was classified as "probably" carcinogenic to humans by the World Health Organization's cancer experts. Scientific research also linked DDT to miscarriages, liver damage, and other health problems, and by 1972 the pesticide once declared a "benefactor to all humanity" had been banned for most uses. Still today, regulatory tests routinely find traces of DDT residues in food.

Don Huber, professor emeritus of plant pathology at Purdue University, believes that glyphosate may be even more toxic than DDT. "Future historians may well look back on our time and write about us . . . how willing we were to sacrifice our children and jeopardize future generations based on false promises and flawed science just to benefit the bottom line of a commercial enterprise," he said. "We need to recognize what the concerns are, what's happening, and then we need to change."[18]

While there is great debate over the safety of glyphosate, there is little doubt about its pervasiveness. By 2013, glyphosate use was so widespread that U.S. government researchers were documenting it in our air and waterways as well as in human and animal urine, including that of dairy cows. An analysis of state water agency data by the nonprofit Environmental Working Group found glyphosate in tap water in at least six states, flowing through water utilities that serve more than 650,000 people. People getting their drinking water from utilities in Bakersfield, California, and New Port Richey, Florida, were among those exposed.[19] Glyphosate residues have also been found by various organizations in a range of commonly consumed products, including wine, cereals, and snacks. Although everyone who eats risks glyphosate exposure, agricultural workers who toil in fields where the pesticide is used face the greatest exposures.

Harrington Investments, a California-based investment advisory firm that focuses on socially responsible investments, believes Monsanto can and should do more to reassess glyphosate's impacts. John Harrington, who leads the firm, has filed multiple shareholder resolutions asking Monsanto's management team to conduct fresh studies on glyphosate's consequences for both people and the environment, but each request has been rejected.

WHAT KILLED JACK McCALL? 21

"They have a long history of egregious behavior," Harrington said about Monsanto. "They operate with no regard for the potential harm that may result from their actions—profit is their sole objective. Monsanto is the quintessential example of a corporation that exists exclusively to maximize materialistic self-interest, regardless of the consequences to society."[20]

~

Jack McCall's death was felt throughout his small community of Cambria, an old mining town at the mouth of the Santa Rosa Creek, midway between the bustling cities of San Francisco and Los Angeles. The community, home to about 6,000 people, is dotted with vineyards and wineries, verdant pastureland, and rolling hills of brilliant yellow flowers, and it is blessed with easy access to the rocky beaches of the Pacific Ocean.

Everyone in Cambria knew Jack, it seemed. He worked for years as a town postman to help make ends meet, volunteered in a local church, and was a fixture at the local farmers' market, where he offered fresh fruit for sale or traded avocados for vegetables to take home for dinner.

Longtime family friend and neighbor Shanny Covey said that while Jack was worried about other pesticides, he believed that glyphosate was safe. He used it over and over and recommended it to Covey and other friends and farmers. He was so confident of the safety of his fields that he would take his grandson Wyatt for tractor rides around the farm. Three years before Jack's death, the McCall family dog, Duke, developed lymphoma and died at the age of six. Duke had typically romped alongside McCall and played in the areas where McCall used glyphosate to treat weeds. But no one suspected at the time that the weed killer could harm the dog.

When Jack was diagnosed with non-Hodgkin lymphoma in 2015, his oncologist warned Teri not to try to research the particularly fast-moving and rare form of NHL Jack had—anaplastic large-cell lymphoma, or ALCL.

The prognosis was so dire it would be better for Teri not to know. Teri did the research anyway.

Some of what she learned, she already knew: ALCL revealed itself slowly at first, with symptoms easy to discount—fever, backache, loss of appetite, and fatigue. It could start in the skin, or the lymph nodes, or in organs anywhere in the body. And it could kill.

"I saw that it was aggressive, but I still was determined that we were going to lick it," she recalled. "He wanted to talk about making plans for me, for the family, in case he didn't make it. But I avoided that. I always thought there would be more time. I didn't know he was dying."

It was Christmas Eve 2015 when Jack was admitted to the hospital for what would be the final time after he suffered a massive stroke. Cancer had spread from an initial lump in his neck throughout his body, and he was weak from chemotherapy and other treatments. His body simply could not take any more. Family and friends gathered at his bedside on Christmas Day to say their goodbyes before Jack slipped into a coma that he would not come back from. He died the day after Christmas when Teri allowed his doctors to remove life support. "I wanted to tell him not to leave me, but I couldn't do that to him," Teri recalled. "I couldn't make it harder for him to go."

Paul McCall, who stepped in to run the farm in his father's place, was the first to make a connection between his father's disease and Roundup, stumbling onto IARC's findings during an Internet search. He read about the strong links found between glyphosate and NHL and read more and more until the rage and grief overwhelmed him. It was too late to help his father. But Paul decided there would be no more Roundup used on the farm. He started warning friends and neighbors about the herbicide as well. He knows his suspicions don't prove the chemical is the killer, but he refuses to take what he sees as more risks. "I threw it all out. I just use dish soap mixed with some vinegar and salt now. It works just as well," he said. "It's no secret Roundup is bad for you. They got rid of DDT. They need to get rid of this too."

CHAPTER 2
An Award-Winning Discovery

It's unclear if Swiss chemist Henri Martin ever fully understood the billion-dollar baby he brought into the world when he discovered what would eventually become known to scientists as *N*-(phosphonomethyl) glycine, or glyphosate.[1] After all, Martin was not looking for an herbicide; he was looking for a drug. It was 1950, the dawn of an era in which efforts to address global health issues were evolving into fresh profit centers that spawned waves of new drug offerings. General scientific research, particularly biological research, was expanding; enhanced mechanization meant faster and more robust production of new drugs; and the race was on to find the latest and greatest magic potion. Martin was working at the time for a small pharmaceutical company called Cilag, which would be acquired by the burgeoning giant Johnson & Johnson Company in 1959.

During long hours in his lab working with different compounds, Martin synthesized a few grams of glyphosate, but the scientist could not come up with any pharmaceutical use for the odorless, crystalline-like substance, and it was ultimately shelved alongside numerous other intriguing but uncertain projects. It would be almost another two decades before any use for glyphosate was found.

After Johnson & Johnson bought Cilag, it sold off several of its research samples, including its glyphosate work, and, like an unwanted stray, glyphosate was sold again by a company called Aldrich Chemical. Stauffer Chemical Company was perhaps the first to find value in glyphosate, identifying it as a chemical chelator, something that could bind with minerals such as calcium, manganese, copper, and zinc. But it took Monsanto Company's chemists to unlock the magic of the molecule as a powerful, and ultimately highly profitable, herbicide.

The glory for that discovery would go to John Franz, a zealous young scientist who would later tell interviewers that he had known he wanted to be a chemist from the age of ten. Franz joined Monsanto in 1955 as his first job after obtaining a doctorate in organic chemistry at the University of Minnesota. He worked on an assortment of projects for Monsanto, which at that time was primarily a maker of industrial chemicals. Franz's work included research into polymer flame retardants.

In 1967, Franz was a fresh transfer into Monsanto's agricultural division, working alongside Phil Hamm, head of the company's herbicide-screening program. The company had been testing different compounds as potential water-softening agents when it found that two molecules showed some herbicidal activity. Weed killers, as well as other pesticides, were in high demand at the time—part of an exploding technology-driven modernization of agriculture and food production. Hamm assigned Franz to analyze these intriguing molecules more closely, and the young scientist ultimately synthesized derivatives into a chemical that could act as a powerful plant growth inhibitor. Glyphosate was considered a novel and highly effective new herbicide. When sprayed on a weed, it travels to the roots and disrupts a critical enzyme produced by plants and microorganisms known as 5-enolpyruvylshikimate-3-phosphate (EPSP) synthase.[2]

Plants require this enzyme to produce the building blocks they need to grow. Without them, the plant withers and dies. Even a few drops of glyphosate can kill an otherwise healthy plant within a few days. In addition to its effectiveness, glyphosate was determined by Monsanto's scientists to be much safer and better for the environment than other herbicides in use. The enzyme glyphosate disrupts was not known to be present in mammals or birds, so while it was toxic to plants, it was safe for people and animals, according to Monsanto.

Monsanto's research team had been searching for nearly a decade for an herbicide that could stop both annual and perennial weeds, so the potential unlocked with glyphosate was quickly embraced by company officials. The first tests of its herbicidal prowess took place in a greenhouse in July 1970 and were so successful that company officials quickly became convinced the discovery could revolutionize the market for herbicides, which had expanded rapidly after World War II. On March 26, 1974, the U.S. Patent Office issued a patent to Franz as the assignor to Monsanto that described the benefits of his invention: "The compositions of this invention provide a wide spectrum of weed control and are also extremely useful as general herbicides as well as in controlling unwanted plants in orchards, tree farms, and various crops."[3]

Franz ultimately found himself showered with awards for his work with the weed killer, including a National Medal of Technology and Innovation bestowed on him by President Ronald Reagan in 1987. Franz told an interviewer for the National Science & Technology Medals Foundation that he found great satisfaction in developing "an environmentally friendly product that's beneficial to mankind."[4] Glyphosate would be later be declared a "one in a 100-year discovery that is as important for reliable global food production as penicillin is for battling disease."[5] Franz was named to the National Inventors Hall of Fame and ultimately would hold over 840 U.S. and foreign patents before retiring from Monsanto in 1991.[6]

～

Franz's discovery came at just the right time for Monsanto. Founded in 1901 by John F. Queeny, the company—named after Queeny's wife, Olga Mendez Monsanto—began as a maker of the artificial sweetener saccharine and then expanded into a chemical manufacturer of everything from sulfuric acid, polychlorinated biphenyls (PCBs), and plastics to synthetic fabrics, expanding its reach over the years with a series of acquisitions.

By the 1940s, the company was one of several in the business of manufacturing the insecticide dichlorodiphenyltrichloroethane (DDT). And in the 1960s, Monsanto became infamous as one of the primary suppliers to the U.S. government of Agent Orange, a defoliant used during the Vietnam War to kill vegetation that provided cover for the enemy. The herbicide, named for the orange-striped drums used to transport it, was a mixture of chemicals called 2,4-D and 2,4,5-T, and military officials asserted for years that the combination posed little danger to people. But Agent Orange was eventually found to contain the highly toxic contaminant dioxin, a by-product created during the manufacturing process that is known to cause cancers and disrupt reproduction and development. Lawsuits and controversy persisted decades after the war ended, with both Vietnamese and U.S. service personnel alleging that Agent Orange caused a litany of ills, including non-Hodgkin lymphoma, prostate cancer, and other diseases. The U.S. government eventually acknowledged the herbicide's role in a wide range of cancers and health problems.

By the 1970s, Monsanto was trying to put the dark cloud of dioxins behind it, and it had an agricultural division under way aimed at adding new herbicides to the company's product line. Weed killers branded with names such as Ramrod and Lasso, invoking images of a toughened cowboy, appeared in the 1960s, and company scientists were racing for more.

When Roundup was rolled out in the 1970s, there was little doubt it would be a hit. Company chemists had combined the active ingredient, glyphosate, with water and the surfactant polyethoxylated tallow amine (POEA) in a formulation that poisoned so effectively that weeds would shrivel and die within days.

Many farmers during that era were using herbicides that formed a chemical barrier on the surface soil of a farm field so that weeds would start dying as they emerged through the ground. But these "preemergent" herbicides washed into streams and groundwater, carrying toxic dangers to wildlife and fish. Roundup was different, according to Monsanto and environmental experts. Evidence showed it was one of the most environmentally friendly herbicides in the history of agriculture, the company assured people.

Monsanto proclaimed that the new herbicide would break down in the soil easily and safely. Glyphosate was also seen as less volatile than other pesticides and less likely to contaminate the atmosphere. And for people and animals, glyphosate was touted as less toxic than aspirin, the company said. Some enthusiastic advocates even proclaimed glyphosate was safe enough to drink.[7] Monsanto itself wouldn't go that far: "Glyphosate isn't a beverage," the company wrote in a blog post. But, it said, "all labeled uses of glyphosate are safe for human health."[8]

Monsanto geared up for high demand of its wonder product, seeking federal approval for expanded mining operations in Idaho of phosphorus—an essential ingredient in its glyphosate herbicides. In applying for the permit, Monsanto told the federal government that production was expected to surge. Monsanto had started mining phosphorus in 1952, at a time when the substance was used mainly in detergents, but by the 1970s it was all about the remarkable new herbicide. The company expected a 50 percent increase in production of the phosphates by 1978, a twofold increase in "about 1981 or 1982," and a threefold increase in production in 1985. At that time, Monsanto was producing at least 220 million pounds of phosphorus in Idaho.[9]

And the company was proved right—the world welcomed its new herbicide. The United Kingdom started using Roundup in wheat production in 1974, becoming the first nation to introduce glyphosate as a tool for food production. In the United States, Roundup initially had been introduced for noncrop uses, and then it was marketed to farmers for use on fields before planting and after harvesting their crops. Malaysia and Canada also quickly adopted Roundup as an answer to weed problems. This was well before the days of the glyphosate-tolerant Roundup Ready crops, which Monsanto developed in the mid-1990s, so farmers had to take care to keep Roundup away from their crops, or they would die alongside the weeds.

The original branded Roundup would be named by *Farm Chemicals Magazine* in 1994 as one of the "top ten products that changed the face of agriculture." Wiping out weeds meant crops had more access to soil moisture and nutrients, which typically translated to higher crop yields at harvest time. But farmers weren't the only ones who loved Roundup. Government agencies that needed to control weeds along roads and rail-road tracks, homeowners, golf course operators, and business park maintenance staff alike were quick to adopt Roundup as their herbicide of choice. The love affair continued well into the new century. As recently as 2008, Stephen O. Duke, a scientist with the U.S. Department of Agriculture's Agricultural Research Service, and Australian weed expert Stephen B. Powles described glyphosate as "environmentally benign," "virtually ideal," and a "once-in-a-century" herbicide.[10]

The writing was already on the wall at that point, as scientific evidence of glyphosate's unintended impacts on the environment and human health was mounting in study after study, but it would not be until 2015 and the World Health Organization's classification of glyphosate as a probable human carcinogen that the world's ardor for glyphosate would turn cold.

There were early warnings, of course, but only a few. The U.S. Environmental Protection Agency (EPA) was still in its infancy back in 1974, when Monsanto marched its new herbicide to the marketplace.

The agency had been created in 1970 by President Richard Nixon as an answer to the environmental movement, an attempt to address American angst over revelations of widespread chemical pollution. Nixon's executive order transferred fifteen units from four other government agencies to form the newly minted EPA. The move wasn't an easy one. Staffers were forced to adjust quickly to new colleagues, nascent policies and administrative practices, and the issuing of literally thousands of new rules and regulations governing the environment. The EPA itself described that early period as "chaos."[11]

Amid the chaos, the new agency was charged with tightening pesticide regulation. Soon, lawmakers passed the Federal Environmental Pesticide Control Act of 1972 to strengthen the severely outdated Federal Insecticide, Fungicide, and Rodenticide Act (FIFRA), which had been passed in 1947 and provided little protection from long-term exposures. The 1972 law moved pesticides from the purview of the U.S. Department of Agriculture (USDA) to the EPA, which was to monitor pesticide residues and strengthen protection of the environment and public health. The idea was to make it easier for the government to ban hazardous pesticides and punish people or companies for improper use.

These directives presented a real challenge to the employees who would oversee the new pesticide registration division, most of whom came from the USDA where a culture of cooperation and affiliation with ag-related corporations was deeply ingrained and there were efforts to promote the advantages of pesticides. After all, part of the USDA's mission was, and is, to support, sustain, and promote the nation's agricultural industry: everyone from small farmers to the giant seed and chemical companies that sell to the farmers.

"These people who came from USDA had very close relations with industry people, the big ag companies," said William Sanjour,[12] who worked at the EPA for thirty years until retiring in 2001. Sanjour was one of a group of EPA scientists who accused EPA officials in the 1990s of failing to investigate allegations that Monsanto falsified scientific studies on the carcinogenicity of dioxin. Monsanto's studies had indicated no link between dioxin and cancer, but the EPA eventually classified the chemical as a "likely human carcinogen."

"They saw the industry people as being their clients—Monsanto, people like that," Sanjour said. "They very much controlled EPA then and they still do." Sanjour won a landmark lawsuit in 1995 against the U.S. government that established the First Amendment rights of federal employees to speak out publicly as whistle-blowers regarding wrongful actions by their employers.

Allegations of collusion aside, regulating pesticides was no easy task, particularly for a new agency that was juggling political and public pressures. It would not be until June 1986—more than a decade after Monsanto's Roundup herbicide was introduced to global markets—that the EPA issued a "registration standard" for the herbicide. And even then, EPA scientists struggled to find consensus, saying additional studies were needed.

The new herbicide was a tough nut to crack. There are actually different "salts" of glyphosate that can be used in different ways in pesticide products. The main one, known as the "isopropylamine salt," is key in controlling broadleaf weeds and grasses in many crops as well as on residential lawns, in forests, and along roadways. It can be formulated as a liquid or a solid and can be applied from the ground or the air. There is also what scientists call the "sodium salt" of glyphosate, used with peanuts and sugarcane to modify plant growth and hasten the ripening of fruit. It is applied as a ground spray to peanut fields and as an aerial spray to sugarcane. The "monoammonium salt" of glyphosate is also used as an herbicide/growth regulator but in only a handful of products.

When the EPA looked at glyphosate in the early and mid-1980s, it determined that many types of additional studies were needed as scientists inside the agency wrestled over the significance of tumors in rats and other health problems seen in test animals exposed to glyphosate. But by 1993, the EPA was trumpeting the safety of Monsanto's herbicide: "EPA's worst case risk assessment of glyphosate's many registered food uses concludes that human dietary exposure and risk are minimal. Existing and proposed tolerances have been reassessed, and no significant changes are needed to protect the public."[13]

The EPA said it had decided to classify glyphosate as a chemical that "shows evidence of non-carcinogenicity for humans—based on the lack of convincing evidence of carcinogenicity in adequate studies."[14] Even though glyphosate would be used by farmers, city workers, homeowners, and others, the agency claimed there was no need for data on occupational or residential exposure because regulators did not have concerns about the chemical's toxicity, especially its carcinogenicity.

But what the EPA did *not* say in that 1993 report was that its conclusion of non-carcinogenicity had actually been a reversal of a prior recommendation by EPA scientists who felt there were noteworthy links between cancer and glyphosate and that the reversal came after prolonged pressure from Monsanto. Critics suspecting collusion demanded to see the data used to justify the EPA's reversal, but for years the agency refused to make public what it said were corporate "trade secrets" that must be protected. Hints of what transpired have recently been revealed in EPA memos that lay out the events and in other documents.[15]

It was February 11, 1985, eleven years after the Roundup herbicide hit the market, when eight members of a group called the Toxicology Branch Ad Hoc Committee of the EPA sat down to consider the carcinogenic potential of glyphosate. The group reviewed a packet of materials that included studies showing links between glyphosate exposure and the development of tumors or other problems in test animals. The group also was given a letter from Monsanto dated February 5, 1985, that sought to discount the significance of the tumors.[16]

One 1983 study stuck out. Several groups of fifty male and fifty female mice, individually caged, were administered diets that included doses of glyphosate for twenty-four months. EPA researchers found results that showed a dose-related increase in incidences of "renal tubular adenomas" in male mice. These kidney tumors were described as a rare type, and the incidence rate seen in the mice exposed to glyphosate, compared with the rate seen in control groups of mice not exposed to the pesticide, could not be ignored. Though adenomas are generally benign— noncancerous—they have the potential to become malignant. Even in noncancerous stages, they can be harmful to many organs. "Review of the mouse oncogenicity study indicates that glyphosate is oncogenic, producing renal tubule adenomas, a rare tumor, in a dose-related manner," a top EPA toxicologist wrote in an internal memorandum.[17]

There were a number of other concerning research results, including another study in which thyroid tumors were observed in some female rats and tumors were noted in the testes of male rats. But the agency showed less concern with those results, concluding that the dose levels in the rat-feeding research were inadequate to assess the chemical's carcinogenic potential for that species. Still, the scientists were worried enough by the kidney tumors in mice that they ultimately determined glyphosate should be considered a Category C oncogen. An "oncogen" is defined as a substance that causes tumors to form. And in EPA lingo, "Category C" translated to "possibly carcinogenic to humans."[18]

That finding did not sit well with Monsanto, and it soon became clear that the 1985 decision was not going to be the end of the discussion. Monsanto continued to protest that links to cancer were unproven and the kidney tumor concerns were unfounded. On April 3, 1985, George Levinskas, Monsanto's manager for environmental assessment and toxicology, noted in an internal memorandum to another company scientist that the company had arranged for Marvin Kuschner, a noted pathologist and founding dean of the medical school at the State University of New York at Stony Brook, to review the kidney tissue slides. Curiously, though Kuschner had not yet even accessed the slides, Levinskas implied in his memo that a favorable outcome from Kuschner's review was ensured: "Kuschner will review kidney sections and present his evaluation of them to EPA in an effort to persuade the agency that the observed tumors are not related to glyphosate," Levinskas wrote.[19]

Levinskas, who died in 2005, was also involved in efforts a decade earlier to downplay damaging findings from a study that found rats exposed to the company's PCBs developed tumors, documents filed in PCB litigation revealed.[20]

Kuschner's subsequent reexamination did—as Monsanto intended—determine the tumors were not due to glyphosate. Looking over slides of the mouse tissue from the 1983 study, Kuschner identified a small kidney tumor in one control group of the mice—those that had not received glyphosate. No one had noted such a tumor in the original pathology report.

The finding was highly significant, as well as controversial, because it provided a scientific basis for a conclusion that the tumors seen in the mice that were exposed to glyphosate were not noteworthy after all. Additionally, Monsanto provided the EPA with an October 1985 report from a "pathology working group" that supported Kuschner's work and also rebutted the finding of the connection between glyphosate and the kidney tumors seen in the 1983 study. The pathology working group said the outcomes reflected a "normal biologic variation" and that "spontaneous chronic renal disease" was "commonly seen in aged mice."[21] Monsanto provided the report to the EPA stamped as a "trade secret" to be kept from the prying eyes of the public.

The EPA's own scientists did not agree, however, saying that additional examination of the tissue slides did not reveal a tumor in the control group. Still, the reports by the outside pathologists brought into the debate by Monsanto helped push the EPA to launch a reexamination of the research. And by February 1986 an EPA Scientific Advisory Panel had dubbed the findings equivocal; the incidences of tumors were not statistically significant enough to warrant the cancer linkage, though the panel did note that "there may be reason for concern."[22] That advisory panel told the EPA that the studies should be repeated in hopes of more definitive findings and that glyphosate should be classified in what the agency at that time called Group D—"not classifiable as to human carcinogenicity." That category was used when the agency determined there was inadequate human and animal evidence linking a substance to cancer or when data were lacking. Later that year, the EPA issued a registration standard that required a range of additional studies to look at toxicology, residues, and environmental issues surrounding glyphosate. The agency specifically asked for a repeat of the mouse oncogenicity study, but Monsanto had no desire to repeat the work and refused to do so. The company argued that "there is no relevant scientific or regulatory justification for repeating the glyphosate mouse oncogenicity study."[23] Instead, the company provided EPA officials with historical control data that it argued supported its attempt to further downplay the tumor incidences seen in the worrisome 1983 study. The company said the tumors in mice appear "with some regularity" and were probably attributable to "genetic or environmental" factors. "It is the judgement of Monsanto scientists that the weight-of-evidence strongly supports a conclusion that glyphosate is not oncogenic in the mouse."[24] After meetings with Monsanto, the EPA's toxicology branch expressed doubts about the validity of Monsanto's data, but eventually EPA officials conceded, stating that they would drop the requirement for a repeated mouse study.

And even though other research acknowledged by the EPA showed apparent ties between glyphosate and blood and pancreatic problems in rats, decreased enzyme production in rabbits, sickness and death in pregnant rats and rabbits, and more, the agency held to a position that there was no significant evidence of danger.

That narrative became so entrenched in the EPA that when a review committee met on June 26, 1991, to again discuss and evaluate glyphosate research, the group decided that there was a "lack of convincing carcinogenicity evidence" in relevant animal studies. The group concluded that the herbicide should be classified far more lightly than the initial 1985 classification or even the 1986 classification proposed by the advisory panel. This time, the EPA scientists dubbed the herbicide a Group E chemical, a classification that meant "evidence of noncarcinogenicity for humans." In a memo explaining the decision, authored by William Dykstra and George Z. Ghali, both scientists within the Health Effects Division of the EPA's Office of Pesticides and Toxic Substances, the agency officials offered a caveat. They wrote that the classification "should not be interpreted as a definitive conclusion that the agent will not be a carcinogen under any circumstances."[25]

Not all the review members agreed with the conclusion in 1991. Of the seventeen peer review members involved, at least two did not concur, writing their objection next to their name. A third simply did not sign the document, which stated "signature indicates concurrence."

Another study examined by the EPA over the course of its glyphosate analysis was one called "A Lifetime Feeding Study of Glyphosate (Roundup Technical) in Rats," prepared by Biodynamics Inc. for Monsanto in 1981. Even though that study showed some tumors in the testes of male rats as well as possible thyroid carcinomas in females who received high doses of the pesticide, it was determined that the data did not demonstrate noteworthy links between glyphosate and cancer. The study was marked by Monsanto as a trade secret and kept from public scrutiny. The 1983 study that showed kidney tumors in mice was also considered a trade secret. In fact, many of the roughly 290 studies, reports, memos, and letters that the EPA said were relevant to its decision making on glyphosate at that time were generated or submitted by Monsanto and were unpublished, meaning they were not peer-reviewed and not available for review or analysis by the public and independent scientists.

The questions about those kidney tumor conclusions have never been fully resolved, at least in the minds of those who believe Monsanto's influence was ultimately what led the EPA to drop its view of glyphosate as a possible carcinogen. The plaintiffs suing Monsanto over cancer claims allege that only scientists with financial ties to Monsanto have ever affirmed the presence of a tumor in the control group for that mouse study. But Monsanto says the evidence overwhelmingly disproves cancer connections.

Some of the research Monsanto provided to the EPA raised red flags in part because fraud had been discovered at two of the laboratories the company used regularly. The deceptions the FDA discovered at Industrial Bio-Test Laboratories (IBT) in 1976 were particularly egregious, leading to the repeat of some toxicology studies of many products, including Roundup. In 1983, three IBT officials were convicted of trying to defraud the government by covering up inaccurate research data. During court proceedings, testimony revealed that IBT laboratory workers sometimes substituted new animals for test animals that had died, without noting the deaths or substitutions in lab reports. Plus, entire test data and lab reports for one product were copied into reports for other products. Then there were the so-called magic pencil studies, in which false data were submitted if test results indicated a product's adverse or fatal effects.

One of those convicted was a Monsanto insider named Paul L. Wright. Wright was a Monsanto toxicologist before he went to work at IBT as a section head for rat toxicology, and he went back to work for Monsanto after the IBT fraud was exposed. He was actually employed by Monsanto at the time he was convicted.[26] Wright also was involved in IBT's testing of PCBs, and memos that came to light during the government's investigation included discussions of efforts by Monsanto to get test results on PCBs altered to cast its product in a more favorable light.[27]

Fraud was also uncovered in 1990 in Craven Laboratories, another lab used by Monsanto to test glyphosate. State and federal investigators found that lab researchers had falsified pesticide residue testing data for at least a decade. Monsanto said that it had all the affected studies done by both Craven and IBT repeated. But critics have little trust in the company-funded reports.

Despite the findings of fraud in the laboratories, it was not easy for the EPA's own experts to challenge companies such as Monsanto. EPA scientist Cate Jenkins, who holds a doctorate in chemistry, found that out firsthand in 1990 when she suspected Monsanto's studies on dioxins were fraudulent and had led the EPA to erroneously conclude that dioxins did not cause cancer. Jenkins alerted top officials within the agency to her suspicions, pointing out "numerous" "misrepresentations and falsifications" in Monsanto's health studies on dioxin submitted to the agency, which made the chemical seem much safer than it was. She accused the company of covering up dioxin contamination problems and engaging in "obvious fraud."[28] Her allegations were shared with Monsanto, which deemed them baseless. In 1991, she pressed the issue again, telling EPA investigators that Monsanto's influence was weakening the EPA's regulation of dioxins. Jenkins was subsequently demoted, an action she responded to by filing a complaint with the U.S. Department of Labor. It took two years of battling for her job before she was reinstated.[29]

Indeed, safety data for pesticides during the era of glyphosate's introduction were so unsound, so suspect, that in a 1982 article in *Mother Jones* magazine, Marcia Williams, former director of the EPA's Special Pesticide Review Division, was quoted as saying that "none of the 600 chemicals which have been registered have adequate data to support them."[30]

Despite the concerns, by September 1993 the EPA had given a green light to Monsanto and glyphosate for a wide range of uses, citing the chemical's safety for humans, animals, birds, bees, and aquatic animals alike. The agency's only noted concern? The "potential hazard to . . . the Houston toad," as the agency stated in a 259-page description of its stance on glyphosate.[31] (The endangered species was facing a host of modern-day development threats, including pesticide use, officials found.)

And in a move that would later fuel criticism, the EPA's safety declarations were largely based on glyphosate alone, not on how it affects people, animals, and the environment when it is mixed with other ingredients, as it is in branded herbicide formulas such as Roundup. Research has shown that these combinations of glyphosate with other chemicals might be more dangerous than glyphosate alone. By 2016, European and U.S. regulatory authorities would be talking about the need to more thoroughly examine these "formulated" products.

"The whole pesticide approval process is so narrowly focused on individual ingredients that no one at the EPA has taken a step back to look at the bigger picture; and when you look at the bigger picture, it's clear that the agency has created a monster," said Nathan Donley, who holds a doctoral degree in cell and developmental biology. "Pesticide labels are so permissive regarding what a pesticide can be mixed with that no one really has any clue about what is being mixed with what and where. The EPA treats pesticide mixtures as something to be swept under the rug. They pay lip service to it every once in a while, but when it comes to actually doing something about it, they revert back to the decades-old practice of pretending that it doesn't exist. With the EPA, lack of evidence of harm equals no harm when it comes to mixture toxicity. It's just indefensible."[32]

One reason for the EPA's apparent eagerness to green-light new pesticides is a little-known provision in the agency's statute that calls for the EPA to examine not only how a pesticide affects human and environmental well-being but also how it affects the financial well-being of agricultural players. As startling as that may be to consumers, it's a fact that protecting public health and the environment is only part of the equation when the EPA decides whether or not to allow pesticides to market. Many people assume the EPA's sole role is to look at potential hazards, health or otherwise, when evaluating pesticides such as glyphosate. But under the law, the EPA must balance risks against benefits, weighing whether or not a pesticide creates an "unreasonable risk to man or the environment, taking into account the economic, social, and environmental costs and benefits of the use of any pesticide." The EPA does a risk-benefit analysis, taking into account that "even though pesticide use entails some risk, pesticides provide substantial benefits to society."[33]

As the agency wrestled over safety concerns with glyphosate, it also was busy figuring out how much of the pesticide would legally be allowed into the food supply. Not coincidentally, many of the studies and reports Monsanto provided to the EPA concerned the fact that using glyphosate in farming was bound to leave glyphosate residues in food. The fact that the agency reversed its earlier view that glyphosate could be a possible carcinogen was key because food safety laws frowned on allowing residues of cancer-causing chemicals in food. By 1991, the company had submitted specific reports aimed at establishing or raising government allowances for glyphosate residues in numerous crops, including corn, soybeans, wheat, potatoes, sorghum, grapes, and dozens of others.[34] Because Roundup was used on tea plantations in Argentina, India, Sri Lanka, Taiwan, and elsewhere, Monsanto even requested allowances for the weed killer in instant tea.[35]

Using Monsanto's work as a guide, the EPA set what the agency calls "tolerances," essentially benchmarks for levels of glyphosate residues that would be permitted on a range of food crops. Those tolerance levels were tied to how much of the chemical was expected to be used on different crops and how much residue was expected to remain. Over the years, Monsanto requested and received approvals for greater and greater tolerances to dovetail with the increasing amounts of its weed killer being used on food and livestock feed crops, setting up the potential for people and animals to consume higher and higher levels of weed killer in their daily diets.

The EPA has made clear that it does not believe these residues pose a threat. The agency states that "the chronic dietary risk posed by glyphosate food uses is minimal."[36] And that belief—the EPA's assurance of safety—was cited for years by other federal agencies as a reason why they skipped over glyphosate when conducting annual testing programs specifically designed to make sure pesticide residues on food were within legal limits. Glyphosate got a pass while other, less widely used pesticides did not. Without such tests, there was no way of knowing if the ever-higher legal levels for glyphosate were being adhered to—or if the food supply was being contaminated with a flood of the weed-killing chemical.

The EPA's flexible allowances for levels of glyphosate residues in food would prove to be critical to Monsanto's future as an agricultural powerhouse. By 1993, Monsanto's patent protection on glyphosate was approaching its sunset—it would expire in 2000 in the United States. After that, rivals would be free to offer cheaper generic glyphosate herbicides to compete with Monsanto's Roundup. But Monsanto had a strategy to keep its Roundup sales strong. The company's scientists had figured out how to alter the genetic makeup of soybeans and other widely grown crops so that they could withstand being sprayed directly with glyphosate. These "Roundup Ready" crops marked the dawning of a new era for agriculture that would quickly and drastically change the face of food production. The EPA's stamp of approval for the safety of Monsanto's Roundup was an essential first step. Monsanto would later cite the EPA's determination that glyphosate did not cause cancer when asking the USDA to approve its new glyphosate-tolerant crops. And by 2001, only five years after the introduction of those Roundup Ready crops, glyphosate would be established as the most widely used agrochemical in America.[37]

CHAPTER 3

The "Roundup Ready" Rollout

Mark Nelson was still a young farmer in the mid-1990s, figuring out the best tools and tactics for coaxing corn, soybeans, and wheat from the farm fields of northeastern Kansas, when he started hearing about a new type of high-tech seed that would soon be for sale. Other farmers Nelson knew were talking about it. So were university extension agents and seed dealers. It seemed everyone was talking about, and waiting for, these special seeds that had been transformed by alterations to their DNA. Through the magic of technology, scientists at Monsanto Company had found they could insert genetic material from a strain of *Agrobacterium* into the chromosome of the soybean, transforming the bean into a crop that could withstand being sprayed with Monsanto's Roundup and still continue to grow and flourish. The company then planted and studied the altered soybean seeds in locations around the United States and in Puerto Rico, Argentina, and Costa Rica through 1991 and 1992, developing a wide range of soybean varieties to commercialize.[1]

This was different from the seed breeding of the past, in which scientists crossbred crop species to obtain desired traits, such as hardier and higher-yielding plants. These new crops contained genetic material that had never naturally made its way into a corn or wheat or soy plant. They were the product of high-dollar laboratories where scientists in lab coats pored over petri dishes, and they were patented by Monsanto. Farmers planting these special seeds would no longer be able to save some of the finished crop and replant the seeds, as farmers had for generations. The seeds for these genetically modified organisms (GMOs) had to be purchased new every year, or Monsanto's patent would be infringed.

With a wife and three young daughters to provide for, Nelson was wary of the hefty price tag attached to the new specialty seeds and the fact that those costs would repeat each season. But as the agricultural community around him quickly embraced them, so did he. The benefits were obvious: while farmers previously had needed to till the soil to disrupt weed growth, rotate the types of crops they planted year after year, and often treat their entire barren fields with various chemicals to kill weeds before planting, the combination of Roundup herbicide and Roundup Ready crops made farming much easier. By itself, Roundup was a godsend to farmers like Nelson, but it couldn't be used once crops emerged from the ground because even a light drizzle of the potent pesticide adrift on a breeze could do great damage to a corn or wheat stalk. With the new types of seeds, the herbicide could be used at will.

"We said yes. The sticker shock was big," Nelson said. "But the weed control was great." Nelson was already a big fan of Roundup herbicide. It knocked out more weed types more effectively than the other types of herbicides Nelson had tried, and he was reassured by the company's assertions that it was better for the environment than rival products. Nelson, who grew up helping his grandfather farm, especially liked that Roundup reduced the need for tilling, a practice known to erode soil and deplete moisture and essential nutrients from the ground. "When it came out, that was all we used," Nelson said of Roundup. "We just used it and used it and used it. We didn't even know what was in it; we never heard the word 'glyphosate.' It was just all Roundup."[2]

It was 1996 when Monsanto unveiled its Roundup Ready soybean. Soybeans were, and are, one of the world's largest sources of plant-based protein, ranking as a top crop for farmers and serving as a key ingredient in many types of food for people, pets, and livestock. Soy is commonly found in infant formula, cereals and crackers, rolls and pastries, and even fruit drink mixes and canned soups. It's often used as a meat extender and found in pork link sausages and luncheon meats. And it's used to make an array of products consumed by vegetarians, such as tofu and soy milk. To put it mildly, Monsanto's introduction of the new soybean spelled a very large market opportunity. And because the soybean was designed to be used in conjunction with Monsanto's branded glyphosate-based Roundup, the profit prospects for the company were enormous.

In seeking government approval for Roundup Ready soybeans, Monsanto again touted the safety of its glyphosate pesticide and made clear that selling the new beans was also about selling Roundup. Farmers buying and planting the new beans could "take advantage of this herbicide's well-known, very favorable environmental and safety characteristics," Monsanto told the U.S. Department of Agriculture (USDA).[3]

The company reminded regulators that "glyphosate is only toxic to plants but not to other living species, including mammals."[4] But because of their tweaked DNA, these new crops would not die even if sprayed repeatedly with glyphosate. The company had discovered organisms that conferred resistance to glyphosate in the sludge-filled waste ponds surrounding its Roundup production plant in Luling, Louisiana.

Monsanto told regulators that its new Roundup Ready system—the herbicide combined with the herbicide-tolerant crops—should save farmers money on fuel, for there would be little need to power up tractors and plow weedy fields. The company also said that the Roundup Ready crop system "may" reduce overall herbicide use,[5] a statement that would prove to be not just wrong but colossally so. Herbicide use actually skyrocketed over the twenty years that followed the introduction of Monsanto's Roundup Ready crops, helping Monsanto reap billions of dollars in herbicide sales, on top of the billions of dollars it made from the specialty seed sales. It was a brilliant move for Monsanto, but it was one that environmentalists, scientists, consumers, and regulators would eventually realize came with devastating costs.

~

The Roundup Ready soybean was only the first herbicide-tolerant crop Monsanto would birth from its laboratories. By the year 2000, only four short years after the first biotech soybean was brought to market, and the year that Monsanto's U.S. patent on glyphosate expired, Monsanto was also selling Roundup Ready corn, cotton, and canola, all genetically engineered to tolerate being sprayed with glyphosate-based herbicides. The company, which at that time was spending around $500 million annually on research and development, had also developed genetic alterations that created insect resistance in corn and cotton, and it was combining the traits into the same seeds.

Monsanto was soon rolling in riches, thanks to farmers' reliance on Roundup and the other glyphosate herbicides Monsanto was selling for use with traditional crops, along with the booming demand for Roundup that accompanied the rollout of the company's Roundup Ready crops. Total company sales were $5.5 billion in 2000, roughly half of which came from sales of Monsanto's glyphosate herbicides. The company bragged to shareholders that it saw an 18 percent rise in the volume of the glyphosate products it was selling just from 1999 to 2000.[6] And, it told them, the global market for glyphosate tripled between 1995, before glyphosate-tolerant GMO crops were introduced, and 2001. Monsanto controlled a dominant 80 percent "or above" of that global market for glyphosate. Executives explained that the gains were in part due to the growing number of acres planted around the world with its genetically altered glyphosate-tolerant crops, which at that time stood at about 118 million acres. "Roundup herbicide is key to our integrated strategy," the company told investors.[7]

In addition to corn, soybeans, cotton, and canola, over the next few years Monsanto would expand its roster of Roundup Ready crops to include alfalfa, a type of hay eaten by livestock, and sugar beets, used widely to sweeten foods and beverages.

The herbicide-tolerant trait was spread throughout the seed market as Monsanto licensed its technology to over one hundred seed companies in the 1990s. By 2013, Monsanto's genetic traits were embedded in more than 90 percent of the U.S. soybean crop and more than 80 percent of American corn.

To ensure that farmers kept using branded Roundup rather than generics on the glyphosate-tolerant crops after glyphosate's patent expired, Monsanto tied a range of incentives and penalties to sales of its products. But the company was so aggressive in its dealings that many customers and competitors cried foul. Critics alleged that Monsanto gained a market monopoly by unfairly blocking rival herbicides from the market and limiting overall competition in violation of antitrust laws. In a class action lawsuit brought against Monsanto in August 2007, Texas Grain Storage, also known as West Chemical & Fertilizer, accused Monsanto of engaging in a "comprehensive anticompetitive scheme" to artificially inflate the prices of Roundup. Roundup held roughly 80 percent of the U.S. agricultural herbicide market at that time—in part, Texas Grain alleged, because the company penalized dealers and wholesalers who sold more than a limited amount of competing generic glyphosate herbicides.[8] Monsanto already was a major supplier of glyphosate to other agrochemical companies, but the company limited the price and the amount that rivals could sell, the lawsuit claimed.

Texas Grain Storage, based in West Texas, was just a middleman, buying and storing Roundup in a stainless steel tank to resell to farmers. But the company said Monsanto kept an iron grip on its dealings, monitoring the level of Roundup that Texas Grain had in storage and requiring Texas Grain to alert Monsanto of all sales of competing glyphosate products.

Other lawsuits made similar accusations, including that Monsanto was using its market power to block rival seed developers from gaining wide distribution for their products, and exploiting that absence of competition by repeatedly raising prices for its specialty seeds. The allegations became part of an antitrust probe by the U.S. Department of Justice and several state attorneys general.[9] Monsanto ultimately altered its contracts, and the allegations faded.

But other problems dogged Monsanto's introduction of the Roundup Ready crops. Since GMOs were first introduced, regulators in the United States, Monsanto's home base, had handled oversight of biotech crops through a three-pronged system of shared responsibilities by the U.S. Environmental Protection Agency (EPA), the USDA, and the U.S. Food and Drug Administration (FDA). Each agency looked at the crops through a different lens, and each ultimately came under withering criticism from both internal government audits and outside environmental and consumer advocates who accused regulators of giving Monsanto far too much leeway.

The U.S. Government Accountability Office, the investigative arm of the U.S. Congress, in a November 2008 report cited several problems with biotech crop regulation. Among the many criticisms, auditors reported that regulators did little to determine whether the "spread of genetic traits is causing undesirable effects on the environment, non-GE segments of agriculture, or food safety."[10]

Many complaints made their way to court. In some cases, the USDA was found to have acted illegally or carelessly in approving crops. In one notable case, a coalition of environmental groups, farmers, and consumers filed suit against the USDA in 2006 for approving Monsanto's Roundup Ready alfalfa without doing the full environmental impact study required by law. The groups argued that the genetically altered alfalfa would likely cross-pollinate with nonmodified crops and contaminate conventional alfalfa supplies. Many overseas markets would not buy GMO alfalfa or other crops, and farmers stood to lose a lot of money in sales if their non-GMO crops were tainted.

Another big concern was the potential for overuse of Roundup herbicide and other pesticides, as farmers, environmentalists, and some government scientists were already starting to document the rise of "superweeds" that had become immune to routine spraying of glyphosate. As farmers struggled to contain the resistant weeds, they dumped more and more herbicides on their fields. This chemical treadmill was harming soil health and the safety of groundwater supplies, critics said.

The judge in the case, Charles R. Breyer of the U.S. District Court for the Northern District of California, agreed with plaintiffs that the law had been broken, and he banned further planting of the GMO alfalfa until the government did a more thorough evaluation. An appeals court upheld the ban. The government essentially dropped out of the case and set about trying to do the analysis the court had found lacking. But Monsanto intervened and succeeded in getting the case in front of the U.S. Supreme Court in April 2010.[11] The high court found in Monsanto's favor in a 7–1 decision. The majority did not disagree that the USDA's Animal and Plant Health Inspection Service (APHIS) had failed to follow the law by neglecting to conduct a full environmental impact study. But, the justices said, the lower court had overstepped in banning further planting of the alfalfa until the environmental impact analysis was completed.

In a sharp dissent, Justice John P. Stevens was harshly critical of the majority's decision to side with Monsanto and lift the ban on the new crop, stating the "environmental threat is novel." In conclusion, he stated:

Confronted with those disconcerting submissions, with APHIS's unlawful deregulation decision, with a group of farmers who had staked their livelihoods on APHIS's decision, and with a federal statute that prizes informed decisionmaking on matters that seriously affect the environment, the court did the best it could. In my view, the District Court was well within its discretion to order the remedy that the Court now reverses. Accordingly, I respectfully dissent.[12]

In a similar case,[13] District Judge Jeffrey S. White of the U.S. District Court for the Northern District of California ruled in 2009 that the USDA violated the National Environmental Policy Act when it approved Monsanto's genetically engineered sugar beets, saying the agency failed to adequately assess the impact the crops would have on the environment. The judge found that Roundup Ready sugar beets "may significantly affect the environment" and encouraged growers to "take all efforts, going forward, to use conventional seed." In an August 2010 ruling, the judge formally revoked approval of the sugar beets and criticized the USDA for "not taking this process seriously."[14] After a legal scuffle over whether or not already planted seedlings would need to be pulled from farm fields, the USDA, under pressure from Monsanto, declared that it would partially deregulate the GMO sugar beets to allow for some production as it prepared the environmental impact statement it was supposed to have prepared years earlier. That final report was published in June 2012, and sugar beets were allowed back on the market.[15] More than 1 million acres of sugar beets are cultivated each year in the United States, and most of this acreage is now planted with the glyphosate-tolerant type.

While these cases dealt mainly with the government's lack of oversight, the complaints foreshadowed a barrage of threats to people and the environment as glyphosate use soared. In 1991, roughly 18.7 million pounds of glyphosate was used on crops in the United States, government figures show. By 2001, the chemical bath had reached roughly 100 million pounds, and by 2015, it had climbed to 286 million pounds.

No herbicide has come remotely close to such intensive and widespread use.

More than half of the glyphosate used worldwide—an estimated 56 percent—was sprayed on genetically altered crops by 2015. Oddly, or perhaps suspiciously, the USDA's public reporting of herbicide and other pesticide use on U.S. farms ended in 2008, and it was left primarily to academic researchers and analysts with the U.S. Department of the Interior to try to keep track of the spread of the chemicals.[16]

"Monsanto was blowing smoke at EPA in claiming that herbicide use would go down," said Charles Benbrook, an agricultural industry consultant who holds a doctorate in agricultural economics and is a former director of the National Academy of Sciences' Board on Agriculture. "Their claim was just laughable."[17]

Even more of the weed killer would likely be drenching U.S. farm fields had Monsanto succeeded with its plans to push an herbicide-tolerant trait into another key crop: wheat, a staple in food products around the globe. Monsanto developed Roundup Ready wheat—in a type called hard red spring wheat, which is typically used to make bread flour—in the early 2000s and sought mightily to bring it to market. But buyers in many foreign countries threatened to stop purchasing wheat from the United States if any biotech wheat was mixed into the market.

"In our opinion, it is unacceptable that a fine commodity is genetically modified just for the purpose of making it herbicide resistant, this does not offer a single advantage to the world," wrote Jef Smidts, a director of a large Belgium-based buyer of U.S. wheat that operated mills across northern Europe, in a 2001 memo to American wheat industry leaders. "Monsanto's marketing research . . . is a joke. GMO wheat for sure will be a market destructor."[18]

American farmers who feared losing export markets also pushed back against Monsanto. The opposition became so fierce that in 2004,

Monsanto ended efforts to commercialize the GMO wheat, though the company said in 2014 it still hoped to bring a GMO wheat to market someday.

Even without the genetic modification, Monsanto still encouraged farmers to spray glyphosate directly on wheat and on a number of other crops that are not genetically altered. The trick, Monsanto told farmers, was to apply the herbicide just days before the crops were to be harvested. Marketing materials put out by the company guide farmers in preharvest treatments of the chemical on not only wheat but also milling oats, barley, peas, lentils, dry beans, and other crops. The idea is both to limit the growth of weeds after the field is harvested and, in some cases, to dry out the crops so they mature more uniformly, which makes harvesting more efficient for farmers. Monsanto recommends that farmers use glyphosate in various ways in conjunction with the production of more than one hundred food crops, according to the EPA.

The result is that glyphosate frequently has been used in various stages in the production of everything from alfalfa to oranges, avocados to apples, grapes to grapefruit. Even U.S.-grown almonds, a common snack for health-conscious people, are treated annually on average with an estimated 2.1 million pounds of glyphosate. Likewise, producers of cherries use an estimated 200,000 pounds of the pesticide annually, according to the EPA's analysis. About 3.2 million pounds are used annually for production of oranges; 1.5 million pounds for grapes; 600,000 pounds for walnuts; 400,000 pounds for pecans; 200,000 pounds for lemons; 100,000 pounds for oats; and 80,000 pounds for avocados.[19]

Still, the largest quantities of glyphosate by far are used on corn and soybeans. The USDA calculated that on average between 2004 and 2013, about 101 million pounds of glyphosate was used each year on U.S. soybean fields alone. Corn crops were sprayed with about 63.5 million pounds. Both estimates were up from a prior analysis that ran through 2011, which pegged average annual soybean use at 86.4 million pounds and corn at 54.6 million pounds.[20]

It's not clear just how much glyphosate residue remains in your salad, sandwich, or snack, largely because regulators have elected for years not to look for glyphosate residues when they do annual testing of pesticide residues in food.

For Mark Nelson, who applies glyphosate routinely to his crops, questions about glyphosate's safety are worrisome, but he is not ready to accept the warnings about cancer. Still, he tries to take every precaution, riding in a tractor with a charcoal-filtered cab and donning safety gear to try to avoid contact with the chemical. "We're careful out here," he said.

Standing in his cornfield on a hot August afternoon, Nelson said he knows the end is coming for glyphosate. Even putting aside the health concerns, weed resistance alone has made this once beloved farm aid less and less effective as the years pass. The rewards will soon no longer be worth the risk. "It's just not working like it used to," Nelson said. "I think eventually it's going to go away."

CHAPTER 4
Weed Killer for Breakfast

For many people, a toasted bagel topped with honey might sound like a healthy breakfast choice. Others might prefer a bowl of oatmeal, corn-flakes, or a hot plate of scrambled eggs. Few would likely welcome a dose of weed killer that has been linked to cancer in their morning meal. Yet that is exactly what private laboratory tests in the United States started showing with alarming frequency in 2014: residues of the world's most widely used herbicide were making their way into American meals.

Testing since then, by both private and public researchers, has shown glyphosate residues not only in bagels, honey, and oatmeal but also in a wide array of products that commonly line grocery store shelves, including flour, eggs, cookies, cereal and cereal bars, soy sauce, beer, and infant formula. Indeed, glyphosate residues are so pervasive that they've been found in human urine. Livestock are also consuming these residues in grains used to make their feed, including corn, soy, alfalfa, and wheat. Glyphosate residues have been detected in bread samples in the United Kingdom for years,[1] as well as in shipments of wheat leaving the United States for overseas markets.[2] "Americans are consuming glyphosate in common foods on a daily basis," the Alliance for Natural Health said in its April 2016 report, which revealed glyphosate residues detected in eggs and coffee creamer, bagels and oatmeal.[3]

In January 2015, an advocacy group called GMO Free USA said tests it ordered showed that Kellogg's Froot Loops cereal contained trace amounts of glyphosate. The group blamed Kellogg Company for "feeding children unlabeled GMOs and toxic herbicides" and called for a boycott of Kellogg.[4] The group also said testing showed glyphosate in PepsiCo, Inc.'s Frito-Lay SunChips snacks. The food manufacturers responded by echoing Monsanto Company's assurances, saying that pesticide residues in food are common and that any glyphosate residues are not at unsafe levels.

Researchers from Abraxis, LLC, a Pennsylvania-based scientific diagnostics company, worked with Boston University on their own testing and reported in 2014 that they found glyphosate residues in 41 of 69 honey samples and in 10 of 28 samples of soy sauce purchased from U.S. grocery store shelves.[5]

One lab, Microbe Inotech Laboratories, was used by several concerned companies and groups for early rounds of glyphosate testing, in part because it was founded by a former Monsanto microbiologist, Bruce Hemming, who had a stellar reputation. Microbe Inotech was small, but it had received government grants to conduct food microbiological research. Moreover, Hemming was a career scientist and entrepreneur as well as a former church missionary with twenty-eight grandchildren, and he had a deep passion for using his scientific skills to help people. Hemming started his lab in 1991, offering microbial and biochemical analyses to a range of companies that wanted tests run on their consumer and industrial products. He was surprised when the interest in glyphosate testing emerged in 2014 and was soon very surprised by the results found in his laboratory, which he operates a mere four miles from Monsanto's massive corporate headquarters in a St. Louis suburb. Hemming knew from his work at Monsanto that glyphosate was not supposed to accumulate in the human body, but his lab detected glyphosate in breast milk samples and a range of other substances submitted for analysis. The shock quickly wore off as Hemming's lab became one of only a few in the United States juggling an influx of testing requests from food companies, public and private researchers, and consumer organizations, all trying to determine how much, if any, glyphosate was present in food, water, and bodily fluids.[6] Hemming's reputation and that of his lab came under sharp criticism, however, by Monsanto and others who said the methodology and results were seriously flawed. Hemming's lab was using a method known as an enzyme-linked immunosorbent assay (ELISA), which the lab said was validated. But critics claimed ELISA was too likely to produce false results to be considered definitive proof of anything.

Rising demand for more and better testing prompted one coalition of scientists and activists, working through what they call the Detox Project, to start offering testing in early 2016 through a laboratory at the University of California, San Francisco, that is registered with the U.S. Food and Drug Administration (FDA). The program was designed for individuals curious to learn if glyphosate is present in their bodies through urine testing, but it quickly expanded to include food product testing, using the more precise and well-regarded method known as liquid chromatography-tandem mass spectrometry (LC-MS/MS).

The Detox Project warns would-be testers that they may not like what they find. The group says this on its website:

Glyphosate is present at all levels of the food chain: in water, plants, animals, and even in humans. Every single study that has measured human contamination with glyphosate has found it. . . .

Despite claims that glyphosate has been widely studied by regulatory agencies and industry, little is known about the health effects of glyphosate-based herbicides at levels found in food or water.

In North Dakota, an agronomist at the state university, Joel Ransom, became so curious about glyphosate residue that in 2014 he ran his own tests on flour samples from the region. North Dakota grows much of America's hard red spring wheat, a type that is considered the aristocrat of wheat and carries the highest protein content of all classes of American wheat. It is used to make some of the world's finest yeast breads, hard rolls, and bagels. But growing the wheat and bringing a healthy crop to harvest is not always easy in a state known for cold and damp conditions. To make harvesting the crop easier, many North Dakota farmers spray their wheat crops directly with glyphosate to help dry the plants a week or so before they roll out their combines. The practice is also common in Saskatchewan, across the border in Canada. So when Ransom ran his tests on flour samples from the area, including flour from Canada, he expected to find some samples with glyphosate. He certainly did not expect all of them to have glyphosate residues. But they did. Ransom reported his findings to the Wheat Quality Council in February 2015, telling the group he was surprised by the results because it was generally believed by agricultural experts that if farmers used glyphosate as instructed, the pesticide's residues should not persist in the grain, let alone in the flour made from it.

Researchers from the U.S. Geological Survey (USGS) have also been on the hunt for glyphosate residues in recent years. As an agency of the U.S. Department of the Interior, the USGS's mission is to provide scientific information about the health of the nation's natural resources. Part of its recent work has been tracking glyphosate use in America and the spread of the pesticide through the nation's waterways, air, and soil.

USGS scientists have found glyphosate and something called AMPA (short for aminomethylphosphonic acid) "widely in the environment," including "commonly in surface waters" and in more than 50 percent of soil and sediment samples and water samples from ditches, drains, large rivers, and streams.[7] The scientists also found the pesticide and the related acid in roughly 30 percent of lakes, ponds, and wetland areas.

"Glyphosate is definitely out there. You see it all the time. Glyphosate and AMPA are pervasive in the environment,"[8] said William Battaglin, a USGS hydrologist and past president of the American Water Resources Association. Battaglin coauthored the 2014 study for the USGS that found glyphosate and AMPA so prominently around the United States.[9]

Measuring residues that include those from AMPA, which is created as glyphosate starts to break down, is critical because AMPA is not just a benign by-product; it carries its own set of concerns, scientists believe. The U.S. Environmental Protection Agency (EPA) did at one time include AMPA residues in calculations when setting a "safe" residue level for glyphosate in food, but it has not done so in recent years, a decision that many scientists believe adds to the hidden danger associated with the pesticide.

It's a shell game of sorts, according to biologist Michael Hansen, who is a senior scientist with Consumers Union and a former member of the USDA's Advisory Committee on Agricultural Biotechnology. By not considering AMPA residues when setting the legally allowed levels of glyphosate residue, Hansen said, the maximum residue limit (MRL), or "tolerance," as the EPA calls it, is functionally made much higher. To put it more simply, by ignoring the residues of the by-product of glyphosate, more glyphosate residues are legally allowed to be considered "safe."[10]

Since at least the 1960s, world food and health experts have sought to gauge how much of a pesticide can be ingested on a daily basis—an "acceptable daily intake" (ADI)—over a lifetime without any noteworthy health risk. U.S. regulators typically use the term "chronic reference dose," but the idea is essentially the same—to establish a limit on how much of a pesticide a given individual can ingest, or be exposed to in a day, without exceeding levels that regulators believe could be of concern. Chronic reference doses are typically based on what animal studies show to be the lowest dose at which adverse health effects caused by a pesticide are seen. The EPA takes the human-equivalent amount of pesticide that harms animals and lowers it significantly in a formula designed to provide protection to human health. That acceptable dose is set at 1.75 milligrams (mg) of glyphosate per kilogram (kg) of a person's body weight per day for Americans. The European Union, in contrast, says the acceptable intake is more than fivefold lower, or 0.3 mg/kg/day.

Separately, many countries also set different tolerance levels for the amount of pesticide residue legally allowed in foods. These MRLs vary for different types of grains and food, and they correlate to the maximum amount of residue that is expected following proper application of whatever pesticide the tolerance is tied to. Tolerances for pesticides may differ depending on the commodity. For example, although the tolerance for the insecticide chlorpyrifos is 1 part per million (ppm) on cherries, it is 2 ppm on radishes. The EPA uses the tolerance levels, together with estimated concentrations in drinking water, to calculate people's high-end dietary exposure to a pesticide based on a typical diet, making sure that estimated exposures do not exceed the ADI, or reference dose.

The United States allows among the highest levels of glyphosate residues, which critics say underscores the level of influence Monsanto has with regulators. They point to 2013, when Monsanto asked for, and received, EPA approval to allow even higher tolerance levels than were already allowed on many foods.[11] Thousands of public comments opposing the move were filed with the agency, but the EPA backed Monsanto's position and responded to critics by insisting that glyphosate's safety was proven, exposures through food and water were low, and worries about ties to diseases such as cancer were unfounded. "EPA has concluded that glyphosate does not pose a cancer risk to humans. Therefore, a dietary exposure assessment for the purpose of assessing cancer risk is unnecessary," the agency stated in a public notice.[12]

Tolerance levels for glyphosate have expanded significantly over the years in several crops. Data compiled by agricultural economist and researcher Charles Benbrook show that tolerance levels for wheat, soybeans, and barley have all been raised to levels much higher than they were twenty years ago. The data make it clear that the more pesticide use the chemical companies promote, the higher the tolerance levels are set by the EPA.

The EPA even has gone so far as to say that safety margins called for by law to protect children from pesticide exposures could be reduced when it comes to glyphosate. The Food Quality Protection Act calls for the EPA to use an extra tenfold (10X) safety factor when assessing exposure risk and establishing allowable levels for pesticide residues in food, unless the EPA determines the extra margin is not necessary to protect infants and young children because the substance in question is so safe. That's exactly what the regulatory agency decided with glyphosate, saying it had adequate data to show that the extra margin of safety for glyphosate could be eliminated.[13] "There is a reasonable certainty that no harm will result to the general population or to infants and children from aggregate exposure to glyphosate residues," the agency stated in its 2013 decision to raise the allowable limits of glyphosate residues in some foods.[14]

Even with the EPA's generous allowances for glyphosate residues, many of the various individuals and organizations doing their own testing have found levels that exceed the tolerances, though many tests do show residues falling within the allowed thresholds. Still, critics say even residues that the EPA says are at safe levels may in fact be harmful to human health when consumed meal after meal, day after day. They believe that the EPA's analysis is outdated and not sufficient to protect people from the pervasiveness of many pesticides, such as glyphosate, that are often combined in food.

Data from animal experiments suggest that when glyphosate is consumed, 15 to 30 percent of it is absorbed into the body.[15] Some research has also shown it can cross the placenta during pregnancy.[16]

But there are far more questions than answers when it comes to glyphosate in food, according to businessman Henry Rowlands, who launched the Detox Project in California to test food and bodily fluids for glyphosate residues. Rowlands, who is from Wales, spends most of his time in Bulgaria, where he owns a language translation business. But his family heritage is rooted in farming, and as he watched the global debate over glyphosate unfold, he jumped in with both feet, getting to know researchers, working with activists, and putting his own money behind efforts to raise awareness. Rowlands said he found quickly that glyphosate is such a hot-button issue that even trying to find independent laboratories to run tests is a challenge. All but two of the American labs he sought out to help launch large-scale testing declined. More than 350 turned him down before Rowlands was able to forge an arrangement with the FDA-registered Anresco Laboratories in San Francisco to offer glyphosate residue testing to both nonprofits and commercial companies.

"I'm certain it was political," Rowlands told me in a call from Bulgaria. "All of these labs test for big food producers. They aren't going to risk their bottom line looking for something food companies don't want people to find. It's really sad. They're not protecting public health." In some of the early work Rowlands had done by Anresco, the lab found glyphosate residues in a range of popular processed foods, including popular brands of cold cereals, crackers, and cookies.[17]

The private and nonprofit attempts to test foods for glyphosate residues were well under way when the World Health Organization's cancer experts made their March 2015 decision to classify glyphosate as a probable human carcinogen. But testing efforts doubled after that, in large part because WHO's decision didn't stand alone; rather, it added to warnings that many scientists had been making for years. The fallout was fast and furious as various government bodies and consumer groups rushed to respond. California's Office of Environmental Health Hazard Assessment (OEHHA) went so far as to issue a public notice in September 2016 that it would list glyphosate as a cause of cancer under requirements of the state's Safe Drinking Water and Toxic Enforcement Act of 1986. In Germany, consumer protection officials called for a ban on glyphosate, and Colombia halted a program encouraged by the United States that sprayed glyphosate on illegal coca fields. Consumer organizations in the United States and Europe demanded that regulators take steps to restrict or ban glyphosate herbicides to protect both human health and the environment, and a petition signed by thousands of Americans was presented to the EPA in April 2016 demanding that glyphosate be revoked in the United States.

Members of a nonprofit called Moms Across America, armed with data about glyphosate residues, boarded a bus and launched a National Toxin Free Town Tour to advocate for a rollback of glyphosate and other chemicals seen as harmful. "The fact is that cities simply cannot afford the risk of using Roundup any longer," said Zen Honeycutt, the group's director. Honeycutt, the mother of three boys, founded Moms Across America after she became convinced that pesticide-laden food contributed to the life-threatening food allergies that plagued one of her young sons. Her group's motto is Empowered Moms, Healthy Kids. Glyphosate is one of the group's most feared foes.[18]

Moms Across America and two other nonprofit groups didn't stop with petitions and marches. They sued General Mills in August 2016, accusing the company of deceptive advertising because some of the company's granola products marketed as made with "100 percent natural whole grain oats" were allegedly found to contain glyphosate residues.[19]

Monsanto has done its best to quell the uproar and to assure consumers and regulators that the pesticide is safe. Monsanto officials have stressed repeatedly that they believe even if glyphosate residues are present in food or beverages, they can't be at levels high enough to be dangerous.

So just how is the public to know if glyphosate residues are common in the food they buy for their families? And if the weed killer is in your food, how high are the levels? If the residues are there, are they at least within the levels set by the EPA as safe? Those should not be hard questions to answer. Indeed, because of the undeniable presence and pervasiveness of pesticides, it has long been the responsibility of the U.S. government to track pesticide levels in food and, importantly, to determine whether residues, if present, are below danger levels. Both the USDA and the FDA have spent decades regularly surveying samples of the American food supply to look at levels of pesticide residues. The testing is critical to protecting public health because a range of health problems are tied to pesticides. Some types, such as popular insecticides, are known to affect the nervous system. Others—like glyphosate—are suspected carcinogens; and others have the potential to cause harmful changes in human hormones. According to the EPA's website, the specific health effects of a particular pesticide depend on the pesticide's toxicity and how much of it is consumed. The EPA also notes that infants and children may be especially sensitive to health risks posed by pesticides.

With all that in mind—and considering that glyphosate has been the most widely used herbicide on the planet, and that it has been the top agrochemical in the United States over several years, and that it is commonly used in food production, and that it is sprayed *directly onto* many types of food crops—one might expect it would be the priority in these residue-sampling programs. After all, regulators routinely have looked for residues of other chemicals used far less in food production.

And yet the truth is this: U.S. regulators have spent decades *not* testing for glyphosate residues. Glyphosate stands out as the one key pesticide that regulators do not look for. Consider the Pesticide Data Program (PDP) that the USDA has conducted since 1991. Each year, the agency collects residue data for hundreds of pesticides in a range of food products. The analysis has even included infant formula and other baby foods, as well as drinking water. The purpose of the program is to "assure consumers that the food they feed their families is safe," according to the USDA. In its 2014 PDP annual summary, for instance, the USDA reported testing for residues of more than 400 different herbicides, insecticides, and other pesticides on food products. But how many tests did they run looking for glyphosate residues? None.[20]

Only one time, in 2011, did the USDA search for glyphosate residues. It conducted what it called a "special project"[21] in which it tested 300 soybean samples taken from twenty U.S. states for glyphosate. More than 90 percent—271 of the samples—carried the weed killer residues. Almost all—287—carried AMPA residues. The USDA said in addition to glyphosate and AMPA, eleven different pesticides were found in the soybeans, but less than 21 percent of the samples contained those other pesticide residues. Glyphosate was by far the most pervasive in the beans.[22] Some thought the results might trigger more testing, but the agency said further testing for glyphosate was not a high priority because the chemical was considered so safe. It also said that while residue levels in some samples came close to the glyphosate tolerance allowed by the EPA, they did not exceed those levels.

The USDA did come close to launching a very limited testing program in the spring of 2017, just as glyphosate concerns were reaching a fever pitch. Documents I obtained from within the agency[23] show a plan to test over 300 samples of corn syrup for glyphosate starting in April 2017. But the agency quietly dropped the plan, with little explanation, just a couple of months before it was to begin.[24]

One of the USDA's excuses for not testing for glyphosate has been cost—the agency has said repeatedly over the years that it is too expensive and inefficient to look for glyphosate residues in food headed for

American dinner tables. And, the agency says, because glyphosate is considered so safe, testing would be a waste of time. That argument mimics Monsanto's own—the company says if the USDA did seek to test for glyphosate residues in food, it would be a "misuse of valuable resources."[25] Yet, while U.S. regulators don't test for glyphosate residues in the foods Americans eat, a division within the USDA known as the Grain Inspection, Packers & Stockyards Administration (GIPSA) does test for the residues in crops headed for food production overseas. GIPSA has been quietly testing wheat for glyphosate residues for years because many foreign buyers don't want glyphosate in this important food crop. GIPSA's testing is part of an "export cargo sampling program," documents I obtained from within GIPSA show. GIPSA's tests found glyphosate residues in more than 40 percent of hundreds of wheat samples examined in 2009, 2010, 2011, and 2012, according to documents I obtained through a Freedom of Information Act (FOIA) request. The levels vary, the data show, ranging up to 10 parts per million (ppm), well above the 4 ppm that Monsanto at one point had told the EPA should be tolerated and considered safe.[26] GIPSA's testing results were not made available to the public in the USDA's annual program reports, however. GIPSA's job is not to report these findings to the public but rather to work with grain handlers, test manufacturers, and life science organizations to help in the marketing of U.S. grain.

The FDA, like the USDA, has spent decades skipping any testing for glyphosate residues, despite the fact that looking for pesticide residues in food is also part of the agency's mandate for public protection. Since 1961, the agency has been conducting what it calls the Total Diet Study (TDS) to monitor levels of about 800 contaminants and nutrients in the average U.S. diet. The agency says that to conduct the study, it buys, prepares, and analyzes about 280 kinds of foods and beverages from representative areas of the country, four times a year. The program began as a way to monitor for radioactive contamination of foods, but over time it expanded to include pesticides, industrial and other toxic chemicals, and nutrients. The FDA also conducts a "residue monitoring program" that measures pesticide levels in thousands of samples of fruits and vegetables as well as other commodities. "The ongoing nature of the study enables us to track trends in the average American diet and inform the development of interventions to reduce or minimize risks, when needed," the FDA states on its website.[27]

But while it has spent years analyzing levels of other types of pesticide residues on food, the FDA, like the USDA, has steadfastly avoided testing for glyphosate residues in the American food supply. Never once, even as glyphosate use on food crops was skyrocketing in the 1980s and 1990s, not even one time, did the FDA look for glyphosate—despite knowing that glyphosate residues were bound to show up in food. Tim Begley, a high-ranking official in the FDA's Center for Food Safety and Applied Nutrition, wrote to Michael Kashtock, another top official in the FDA's food safety office, in January 2013 about illegal uses of glyphosate in Canada, Mexico, Thailand, and Brazil on "some grains, soybeans, citrus, tropical fruits including mangoes." The European Union found a "hit rate" of about 10 percent in cereals, Begley wrote. The agency should start developing a method so that at some point it could test for glyphosate, he said.[28]

Still, it was only in February 2016, nearly a year after WHO's classification of glyphosate as a probable human carcinogen, and with public pressure mounting for government accountability, that FDA officials said they would do some *limited* testing for glyphosate residues on a handful of foods that included corn, milk, and eggs. And that was nearly two years after the U.S. Government Accountability Office (GAO) sharply rebuked the agency for its failure to look for glyphosate. In its 2014 report, the GAO also hammered the FDA for not telling the public that it was skipping over glyphosate testing. And—in a worrisome note—the GAO also made clear that even if the FDA had been testing, there was no surety the results would be reliable because the agency's practices were deeply flawed. According to the criticism leveled by the GAO, there were significant limitations to the credibility of the FDA data on chemical residues that the agency did look for. "FDA's ability to reliably identify specific commodities that may be at high risk of violating pesticide residue tolerances is limited," the report stated.[29]

In its defense, the FDA cited the costliness of testing for glyphosate, just as the USDA had done. The start-up costs for glyphosate testing at six FDA testing laboratories would be around $5 million, according to a statement the FDA gave the GAO.

Considering the stakes, not to mention the fact that the FDA's federal budget is around *$5 billion,* the excuses and inaction frustrate many moms, such as Laura Bowman of Scottsdale, Arizona. Bowman is not a member of any of the burgeoning "food movement" organizations that have sprung up in recent years, but she does consider herself fairly well educated on the dangers of pesticides and other chemicals, and she does her best to protect her family from them. She banned the use of Roundup to control weeds in her yard long before the recent controversies flared, but she feels it's nearly impossible to keep glyphosate out of her family's meals. "I feel like it's in almost everything we consume and our kids consume . . . and the frustrating part is our government does nothing about it," said Bowman, who tries to serve organically grown foods to her husband and two daughters whenever possible in an effort to minimize consumption of pesticide residues. "You try to do the small amount you can do, but so much of it is out of our control."[30]

Canadian authorities also ignored glyphosate in annual residue testing for years, but after WHO's glyphosate classification they jumped into action, and in early 2017 the Canadian Food Inspection Agency (CFIA) announced the results: with a little more than 3,100 foods tested for glyphosate, residues of the weed killer were found in roughly 30 percent of the samples. The CFIA assured consumers there was nothing to worry about because only 1.3 percent of the samples showed residues above the tolerance levels. Still, the results were upsetting to many. Roughly 4 percent of the grain products tested had such high levels of glyphosate that they violated legal limits, the CFIA report showed.[31]

It's not just glyphosate residues that people worry about, of course. Fears about a range of chemical residues in food have been growing in recent years. Pesticide residues can be found in everything from mushrooms to potatoes and grapes to green beans. One sample of strawberries examined by the USDA in an annual testing program found residues of twenty pesticides in the berries. In fact, roughly 85 percent of more than 10,000 food samples tested by the USDA in 2015 carried pesticide residues. Most of those foods were fruits and vegetables, both fresh and processed—foods consumers generally consider healthy. Residue levels higher than what the government allows have been found in spinach, strawberries, grapes, green beans, tomatoes, cucumbers, and watermelon. Even residues of chemicals long banned in the United States were found as recently as 2015, including residues of DDT or its metabolites found in spinach and potatoes.[32] U.S. regulators have also reported finding illegally high levels of the neonicotinoid insecticide thiamethoxam in rice.

The USDA asserts that all these pesticide residues are nothing for people to worry about. The agency states that "residues found in agricultural products sampled are at levels that do not pose risk to consumers' health and are safe."[33] But many scientists say there is little to no data to back up that claim. The animal studies the regulators rely on to set the allowable pesticide levels are typically conducted by, or on behalf of, the pesticide companies and look only at the effects of one pesticide at a time. Regulators do not have sufficient research regarding how consuming residues of multiple types of pesticides affects us over the long term, and government assurances of safety are simply false, say the skeptical scientists.

"We don't know if you eat an apple that has multiple residues every day what will be the consequences twenty years down the road," said Chensheng Lu, associate professor of environmental exposure biology at the Harvard T.H. Chan School of Public Health. "They want to assure everybody that this is safe, but the science is quite inadequate. This is a big issue."[34]

When it comes to pesticide exposures, through food or otherwise, researchers are particularly worried about children. Multiple studies suggest pesticides are harming children's brains and bodies. Researchers found that women's exposure to pesticides during pregnancy, measured through urine and blood samples, was associated with negative impacts on their children's IQ and neurobehavioral development, as well as with attention deficit hyperactivity disorder diagnoses.[35] Also, one study that looked at structural brain growth using magnetic resonance imaging found "significant abnormalities" in measurements of the brain and determined that children whose mothers were exposed to organophosphate pesticides showed neurotoxic effects well into the early school years, at least.[36]

A team of international scientists examining the effects of pesticides in food and on farms summed up the problem this way:

> Recent insight into the toxic effects of pesticide exposure suggests that early-life exposure is of greatest concern, especially prenatal exposure that may harm brain development. . . . No systematic testing is available since testing for neurotoxicity—especially developmental neurotoxicity—has not consistently been required as part of the [regulatory] registration process. . . . At least 100 different pesticides are known to cause adverse neurological effects in adults, and all of these substances must therefore be suspected of being capable of damaging developing brains as well.[37]

Philippe Grandjean, a coauthor of that report and a Harvard adjunct professor of environmental health who received his medical degree in Denmark at the age of twenty-three, believes the warning signs must be taken seriously. He urges women who are pregnant, who plan to become pregnant, or who are breastfeeding to seek out organically grown foods because their pesticide levels are far less than those found in conventionally grown foods. Grandjean is an expert in this area, traveling the world to study environmental problems and to examine children whose lives have been affected by environmental chemicals. He received the John F. Goldsmith Award from the International Society for Environmental Epidemiology in 2016 for "sustained and outstanding contributions to the knowledge and practice of environmental epidemiology."

"Overall, consumption of organic food substantially decreases the consumer's dietary pesticide exposure, as well as acute and chronic risks from such exposure," the scientists' report stated. "Pesticides undergo a comprehensive risk assessment before market release, but important gaps remain."[38] Grandjean has little faith in regulatory assurances that current limits on pesticide amounts in certain foods are safe. "Those limits are based on animal studies, looking at the effect of one pesticide at a time," he said. "The human brain is so much more complex than the rat brain, and our brain development is much more vulnerable."[39]

Though pesticide residues are invisible, odorless, and tasteless, more consumers are becoming aware of—and unsettled by—their presence. Every year for the past decade, the International Food Information Council (IFIC) has surveyed more than 1,000 Americans to gain insight into their attitudes toward food and diet. The group, which quizzes people ranging in age from eighteen to eighty, says the results show a clear and steady rise in the number of Americans concerned about chemicals in their food. More than one-third of consumers participating in an annual food industry survey in 2015 and 2016 rated chemicals in

food as their most important food safety issue, and many report changing their eating habits because of their worries.[40]

But glyphosate stands out as among the most feared, largely because it
is so pervasive, because there are ongoing questions about its safety, and
because of the government's reluctance to monitor foods for glyphosate
residues. With all that in mind, the recognition that this weed-killing
pesticide is in our food is more than many can stand. San Francisco resident Danielle Cooper filed a lawsuit in April 2016 seeking class action
status against the Quaker Oats Company after glyphosate residues were
found in that company's oat products, which are used by millions of
consumers as cereal and for baking cookies and other treats. Cooper said
she expected the oat products, labeled "100% Natural," to be pesticide
free. "Glyphosate is a dangerous substance, the presence and dangers
of which should be disclosed," the lawsuit stated.[41] Quaker, owned by
PepsiCo, responded to the lawsuit by saying that glyphosate residues, if
present, were so low as to not be a problem.

Worries about weed killer residues have also disrupted international
trade. In May 2016, Taiwan authorities and U.S. food safety inspectors
found glyphosate residues in oatmeal products imported by Taiwan,
prompting a recall of nearly 62,000 kilograms of oatmeal.[42]

The concerns in the marketplace finally prompted one of the FDA's
most talented chemists, Narong Chamkasem, to run his own in-house
tests on glyphosate in oats. Chamkasem had obtained a doctorate in
analytical chemistry and worked for the giant Swiss agrochemical company Syngenta AG for fifteen years before joining the FDA in 2008,
and he was quite familiar with the ins and outs of testing for agrochemicals. At that time, FDA scientists were working to bring the agency
into the modern era of pesticide residue testing, implementing methods
that were already in place in Australia, Canada, China, Denmark, Germany, Japan, the Netherlands, and the United Kingdom. Because the
FDA had not looked for glyphosate residues in food for decades, the
tests Chamkasem ran on oats were among the first. The results were not

reassuring for anyone worried about feeding themselves or their children. Just as did the private researchers, Chamkasem found glyphosate residues in numerous oatmeal products, including infant oat cereal. He presented his findings to a group of chemists in a meeting in Florida in July 2016, but the FDA did not publicize the findings at all.

Oats are not genetically engineered to tolerate glyphosate. But Monsanto has encouraged farmers to spray oats and other non–genetically modified crops with its glyphosate-based Roundup herbicides shortly before harvest to help dry down and even out the maturity of the crop. The company even provides farmers with a booklet telling them: "A pre-harvest weed control application is an excellent management strategy to not only control perennial weeds, but to facilitate harvest management and get a head start on next year's crop."[43]

In Canada, which is among the world's largest oat producers and is a major supplier of oats to the United States, Monsanto marketing materials tout the benefits of glyphosate on oat fields: "Preharvest application of Roundup WeatherMAX and Roundup Transorb HC are registered for application on all oat varieties—including milling oats destined for human consumption."[44] Glyphosate is also used by U.S. oat farmers. The EPA estimates that about 100,000 pounds of glyphosate is used annually in production of oats in the United States.

Considering the growing public angst over pesticide residues in our food, one might have expected FDA officials to shout it from the rooftops when the agency decided to start a formal glyphosate residue testing project in 2016. That was not the case. The agency made it clear that until the results were in, the less that was publicly known about what it was doing, the better. I got wind of the FDA's decision to do at least one glyphosate residue testing project through a couple of government sources who couldn't talk to me about it openly because they said the issue was so "sensitive." It took weeks of badgering before the FDA would even acknowledge to me that it planned to do some tests for glyphosate. I wrote a news story[45] about that move that got picked up and repeated around the world, but FDA officials repeatedly refused to answer many important questions about the methodology and whether or not Monsanto had any influence in the testing project. The agency also balked at producing documents about its glyphosate residue testing work. Among the documents it did produce as a result of my FOIA requests, many contained heavy redactions, meaning many sections were blacked out.

What was revealed in these pages, however, was concerning enough. Take honey, for instance. Again, it was Chamkasem doing the work. According to those FDA documents,[46] when Chamkasem examined honey samples from various locations in the United States, he came up with alarming results: he found that all of the honey examined, including "organic" honey, contained glyphosate residues. Some of the honey even showed residue levels more than five times the legally allowed limit in the European Union, according to these internal documents and research data. One brand that contained the residues was Iowa-based Sue Bee Honey, which is marketed by a cooperative of American beekeepers as "pure, all-natural" and "America's Honey." One sample of honey from Iowa showed glyphosate residues at 650 parts per billion (ppb), well over the 50 ppb allowed in the European Union.

Now, honey comes from bees, of course, and beekeepers do not use glyphosate on their hives. There is no need, as weeds are not an issue in beekeeping. But bees travel many miles, and when they are near farm fields, they spend their days darting from plant to plant, including an array of crops such as cotton, alfalfa, soybeans, and many others grown in fields that are sprayed with glyphosate. The pesticide travels back with the bees to the hives, where the honey is produced. Darren Cox, past president of the American Honey Producers Association, describes bees as "flying dust mops," picking up everything they touch. With that in mind, it's easy to see how glyphosate levels might be high in honey from Iowa, given that Iowa is the nation's top corn-growing state and most of the corn is genetically modified to be sprayed directly with glyphosate.

When Chamkasem found such high levels in honey, he wrote to colleagues in January 2016 e-mail exchanges, notifying them of his findings and pointing out that at that time there was no legal tolerance level for glyphosate in honey in the United States, so any amount of detectable glyphosate in honey would be illegal.

True, noted Chris Sack, an FDA chemist who oversees the agency's pesticide residue testing and is considered the agency's "residue expert." But Sack tried to diffuse Chamkasem's concerns: "Before you pursue the regulatory status of honey, you need to know that the agency is undecided about how to address 'violations' of glyphosate in honey," Sack said in the e-mail exchange. "EPA has been made aware of this problem" and was expected to set tolerance levels for honey, Sack wrote. Once tolerance levels are set by the EPA—if they are set high enough—the residues are no longer considered illegal.[47]

Still, the business owners who keep the bees and sell honey are worried. They say it is frustrating to know they can't keep their product free of a pesticide that they have no use for and don't benefit from in any way. Many fear that if public awareness of pesticide levels grows, imported honey from countries that are not so reliant on pesticides will knock them out of the marketplace.

"I'm an innocent man with thousands of beehives. I can't do anything about the farmers using Roundup and the bees picking it up off cotton or something," said Nate Carmichael, a young husband and father who, along with his wife, Marcela, tends to about 10,000 hives and makes a living selling honey to grocery stores and outlets such as Walmart. The company packs around 1 million pounds of honey to sell in a good season. "I don't understand how I'm supposed to control the level of glyphosate in my honey when I'm not the one using Roundup. It's all around me," Carmichael said.[48]

Marcela is a registered nurse who works with oncology patients, and she has long feared the adverse effects that pesticide residues could have on her family's health. She tries to buy organically grown food and feeds her young daughter the healthiest meals she can, so she was shocked and saddened to learn of the weed killer found in her company's honey. "What can you do? I'm sure you'll find pesticides in almost everything. It makes you feel so helpless," she said. "How do we protect our children?"[49]

Knowing that glyphosate is in honey also upsets Margaret Lombard, chief executive officer of the National Honey Board, which promotes honey products to consumers. She sees the situation as not only an injustice to beekeepers but also an indicator of how hard it is to escape contamination of the larger food supply. "It seems like everything we're eating has this chemical in it," she said.[50]

The FDA's decision to start testing for glyphosate residues attracted Monsanto's attention, as would be expected. As testing was ramping up in the spring of 2016, Monsanto's international regulatory affairs manager, Amelia Jackson-Gheissari, asked Lauren Robin, chief of the FDA's Plant Products Branch, to set up a time to talk about "enforcement of residue levels in the USA, particularly glyphosate," according to the FDA records I obtained.[51] The FDA said it does not have extended communications with Monsanto on this topic and Monsanto does not influence the FDA's work. But it's noteworthy that even as the FDA engaged in conversation with Monsanto about residues, it did not inform the public about the glyphosate residues found in honey or in oats.

It's clear the government has long been aware of glyphosate residues in food—in one intra-agency e-mail exchange in 2015, FDA chemist Chamkasem said: "I believe we will see a lot of violation for glyphosate."[52] Within a few months after Chamkasem did his tests, the FDA abruptly halted his pesticide residue testing operations, deciding that additional work could and should be handled by other FDA chemists elsewhere. The FDA also suspended glyphosate residue testing for nine months, resuming limited testing in June 2017.

The fact that the FDA and the USDA have dragged their feet on testing for so long frustrates many who are concerned about the pesticide.

"There is no sense of urgency around these exposures that we live with day in and day out,"[53] said Jay Feldman, executive director of Beyond Pesticides, whose organization met with the EPA in January 2016 to argue for more government action on glyphosate.

The reluctance of the U.S. government to examine food for glyphosate residues has also been noted across the Atlantic, in Europe, where glyphosate is a growing concern. Michael Antoniou, a molecular geneticist in London who has been among many researchers studying glyphosate and formulations such as Roundup, said, "With increasing evidence from laboratory studies showing that glyphosate based herbicides can result in a wide range of chronic illnesses through multiple mechanisms, it has become imperative to ascertain the levels of glyphosate in food and in as large a section of the human population as possible."[54]

CHAPTER 5
Under the Microscope

So just how dangerous is glyphosate? Most people would agree that, as with virtually any pesticide, it's not a good idea to drink it, bathe in it, or inhale it. Farmworkers are trained to wear protective gear when applying or mixing their farm chemicals and to follow an assortment of guidelines to protect themselves and others from harmful exposures. But the question of exactly how dangerous long-term use of glyphosate might be, especially in formulations such as Roundup, has thus far been hard to answer.

Monsanto Company and many leading chemical industry experts tell us that we should trust them and that more research is not needed. The safety of glyphosate and Roundup is proven, they say. But trust is hard to come by when the government does not require robust long-term safety data for a finished product such as Roundup, only for the active ingredient. There have long been concerns that the end product is more dangerous than glyphosate alone, and scientists say it is well-known that extra ingredients in pesticide products not only may themselves be toxic but also may enhance or supplement the toxic effects of the active ingredient. Extra ingredients in pesticides commonly include surfactants that help chemicals stick to the leaves of plants, antifoam compounds, and more. Yet the bulk of industry-sponsored toxicology tests are done using only the active ingredient. As well, there is very little long-term epidemiology data on glyphosate exposure, and there is no established base of information about just how much of the pesticide is in the products we eat and drink because the U.S. Food and Drug Administration (FDA) and the U.S. Department of Agriculture (USDA) have so steadfastly avoided including glyphosate in their testing regimes. And despite industry assurances of safety, there is an international body of published research that contradicts those claims. Several different scientists in several different countries have found associations between glyphosate and disease, most notably a link with non-Hodgkin lymphoma, while independent research on formulated products such as Roundup has found that the combinations of chemicals can be even more hazardous than glyphosate by itself.

In study after study, exposure to glyphosate or Roundup has left laboratory rats and other experimental animals with a range of health problems, including tumors, blood and pancreatic problems, and liver and kidney troubles. Some research showed that exposed male mice developed a sarcoma that started in the lining of their blood vessels, while other work found that glyphosate produced fetal malformations in lab animals. One group of Brazilian scientists found that Roundup appeared to disrupt male reproductive functions by triggering cell death in rat testes.[1]

A team of British scientists that included Michael Antoniou made headlines in early 2017 with the publication of research linking Roundup to fatty liver disease. The scientists mixed low doses of the weed killer with water and then gave the solution to female rats over a two-year period. The dose was about the same as concentrations found in tap water, according to the scientists, and was actually far lower than the levels found in some foods. At the end of the study period, the researchers examined the organs of the animals and found cell damage and clear evidence of disease.[2] Monsanto rejected the findings, as it had with other studies that link glyphosate with disease, saying they were based on flawed data and conducted by agenda-driven scientists. But others saw it as evidence that Roundup was much more harmful than anyone had realized.

Concern grew when a group of Brazilian scientists published research in February 2017 showing that very young lab animals given soy milk laced with glyphosate suffered damaging hormonal changes. The finding raised alarm because mothers often feed soy formulas to their babies as an alternative to breastfeeding, and soy is commonly found to contain glyphosate residues.[3]

Well before that work, molecular biologist and neuroscientist Andrés Carrasco at the University of Buenos Aires and a group of colleagues set alarm bells ringing across Argentina with a 2010 study that found injections of a very low dose of glyphosate into frog and chicken embryos could cause spinal defects. Carrasco's work indicated that glyphosate changed levels of retinoic acid, considered fundamental for protecting the body from cancers and for helping embryonic cells develop properly. Those chicken and frog embryos subjected to heavily diluted Roundup showed serious malformations and/or died.[4] Carrasco, who was a principal investigator at his university's Institute of Cellular Biology and Neuroscience when he did the research, was quoted in an Associated Press story in 2013 explaining that his investigation was triggered by reports of increasing birth and spinal defects in farming communities after crops genetically modified to be sprayed directly with glyphosate were approved for use in Argentina. "If it's possible to reproduce this in a laboratory, surely what is happening in the field is much worse," Carrasco told the Associated Press. "And if it's much worse, and we suspect that it is, what we have to do is put this under a magnifying glass."[5] Carrasco died in 2014, but his findings have left lingering questions for health officials in Argentina.

In Sri Lanka, scientific studies have suggested that a deadly chronic kidney disease that has afflicted thousands of people in farming areas is tied in part to exposure to pesticides, including glyphosate.[6] Both Sri Lanka and El Salvador at one time debated a ban on glyphosate because of fears the chemical could be contributing to the epidemic of the new form of chronic kidney disease, which could not be attributed to diabetes, hypertension, or other known triggers. The World Health Organization became so concerned that it funded a study in conjunction with the National Science Foundation of Sri Lanka to delve into the matter. The resulting research report, published in 2013, surmised that a combination of harmful heavy metals and pesticides could be to blame. Glyphosate residues were among the pesticide residues found in the urine of the kidney patients. Also found was cadmium, a highly toxic metal known to cause cancer.[7] Cadmium is particularly harmful to humans; it targets the body's cardiovascular, renal, gastrointestinal, neurological, reproductive, and respiratory systems.

Sri Lankan toxicologist Channa Jayasumana theorized that glyphosate is a key culprit in the kidney disease seen among agricultural workers not just in Sri Lanka but in other countries as well. According to Jayasumana, a member of the Faculty of Medicine and Allied Sciences at Rajarata University of Sri Lanka, glyphosate's ability to act as a "chelator," a substance that creates bonds with heavy metals, was causing dangerous compounds that could make their way into food and water and eventually reach a person's kidneys. Glyphosate was actually patented as a chemical chelator in 1964 by Stauffer Chemical Company, though Monsanto has argued it is not very potent in that role.[8] One of Jayasumana's research papers explained it this way:

Here, we have hypothesized the association of using glyphosate, the most widely used herbicide in the disease endemic area and its unique metal chelating properties. The possible role played by glyphosate-metal complexes in this epidemic has not been given any serious consideration by investigators for the last two decades. Furthermore, it may explain similar kidney disease epidemics observed in Andra Pradesh (India) and Central America. Although glyphosate alone does not cause an epidemic of chronic kidney disease, it seems to have acquired the ability to destroy the renal tissues of thousands of farmers when it forms complexes with a localized geo environmental factor (hardness) and nephrotoxic metals.[9]

Research also suggests that glyphosate harms human health by exacerbating the damage done by other food-borne chemical residues and environmental toxins. The harm manifests slowly over time, creating conditions that damage cellular systems throughout the body, this theory goes. Some studies have shown that the weed killer is genotoxic, causing DNA damage in human cells that can lead to cancer. Other research indicates glyphosate may harm beneficial gut bacteria needed for healthy immune function.

Many researchers fear that one of the worst impacts of glyphosate on human health may be as an endocrine disruptor, a dreaded term for chemicals that interfere with hormones in the human body in ways that can cause cancerous tumors, birth defects, and other developmental disorders. Endocrine disruptors have been associated with developmental and learning disabilities in children, attention deficit disorder, and cognitive problems.

Humans are very sensitive to very low dosages of endocrine disruptors, according to Andrea Gore, professor and Vacek Chair of Pharmacology at the University of Texas at Austin—especially developing fetuses, infants, and children. "Small fluctuations from the norm can change developmental processes and lead to a dysfunction at the time of exposure, or sometimes, many years after exposure," Gore said in an interview with *Vice* magazine for an article about glyphosate.[10]

Several recent studies have shown the potential adverse health effects of glyphosate as an endocrine disruptor, including the 2017 soy milk study and a 2013 study by a team of four toxicology experts from Thailand who found that glyphosate induced human breast cancer cell growth. "These results indicated that low and environmentally relevant concentrations of glyphosate possessed estrogenic activity," the scientists concluded.[11] A 2009 study by French researchers similarly found that glyphosate-based herbicides triggered endocrine disruption in human cells even at low levels. The scientists warned that the "real cell impact of glyphosate-based herbicides residues in food, feed or in the environment" warranted greater consideration.[12] Another study by French researchers, published in 2016, reiterated that warning, finding that glyphosate-based herbicides such as Roundup have endocrine-disrupting effects at concentrations well below those used by farmers.[13] Scientists have found indications that Roundup and other glyphosate-based weed-killing products induce cell-cycle dysregulation, a hallmark of cancer, and that Roundup can be toxic to human umbilical, embryonic, and placental cells.[14]

One study looking at several communities exposed to glyphosate-based formulations found chromosomal damage in blood cells, and scientists said the markers of chromosomal damage were significantly greater after exposure than before exposure in the same individuals.[15] In a report issued in October 2016, Pesticide Action Network (PAN) International stated:

> Exposure to glyphosate-based herbicides, even at very low doses, may result in reproductive problems including miscarriages, pre-term deliveries, low birth weights, and birth defects. Laboratory studies have shown that very low levels of glyphosate, Roundup . . . and the metabolite AMPA all kill human umbilical, embryonic, and placental cells. Roundup can kill testicular cells, reduce sperm numbers, increase abnormal sperm, retard skeletal development, and cause deformities in amphibian embryos.[16]

One study of pregnant women in an Indiana obstetric practice found glyphosate in the urine of over 90 percent of women tested, and it determined that women with higher levels of the pesticide were found to have shorter pregnancies and babies with lower birth weights, outcomes that are believed to translate to long-term health problems.[17]

Part of the difficulty in establishing clear evidence is the rather obvious fact that researchers cannot ethically use people in experiments with glyphosate, so animal studies and observational studies of the health of people who work in agriculture, spraying crops with Roundup or otherwise being exposed, are the key ways scientists examine the issue. And because the government does not track or collect data on glyphosate residues in food, scientists cannot quantify how that route of exposure corresponds with or affects incidences of disease.

Then there is the problem of trying to identify one pesticide among many that may be the cause of a specific disease. People, particularly farmers, are often exposed to multiple pesticides during their lives, and many pesticides are frequently used together or at least during the same season. Research shows there have been increases in the global incidence of non-Hodgkin lymphoma (NHL) over the past thirty years,[18] and even though the rate has leveled off in the United States recently, it is the seventh most common type of cancer in the United States.[19] Farmers are at increased risk for the deadly cancer,[20] and pesticides are thought to be the chief culprit. But trying to decipher which pesticide or pesticides might be behind the cancer cases has proven challenging.

During the 1980s, the National Cancer Institute conducted three case-control studies of NHL in Nebraska, Kansas, and Minnesota and Iowa—all top U.S. farming states. The Heartland produces millions of bushels of wheat, corn, and soybeans every year, and an array of agrochemicals are used widely. Glyphosate is a favorite. Researchers later pooled the data to examine how the pesticide exposures affected a farmer's risk for the blood cancer. Researchers looking at forty-seven different pesticides found that glyphosate and at least eight other "potentially carcinogenic" chemicals used by the farmers showed links to NHL.[21]

Researchers also found an association between glyphosate and NHL in a separate, much smaller study from 1999.[22] And a 2001 study across a large region of Canada found that the more often people used glyphosate, the higher was their risk for NHL.[23]

There is also fear that glyphosate can be extremely harmful even in low amounts, such as traces of it in our food. By February 2016, around the same time the FDA was saying it would finally start limited testing for glyphosate residues in food, fourteen scientists from Europe, Canada, and the United States issued what they called a "Statement of Concern . . . directed to scientists, physicians, and regulatory officials around the world."[24]

In the statement, published in an open-access scientific journal, the scientists pointed out that to accommodate the increased use of glyphosate that came with Monsanto's rollout of its glyphosate-tolerant crops, regulators "dramatically increased" tolerance levels allowed in corn, soybeans, and other crops. Human exposure has been rising, while regulatory estimates about what a "tolerable" daily intake means for people consuming glyphosate residues is based on outdated science, the group said. The scientists said that research shows low levels of these herbicides can do damage to people in the range of what regulators consider safe, and they recommended that regulators reexamine the acceptable daily intake for glyphosate, which is established at 1.75 milligrams (mg) of glyphosate per kilogram (kg) of a person's body weight per day for Americans but is set much lower in the European Union, at 0.3 mg/kg/day.

The scientists also said that U.S. regulators must prioritize glyphosate for government-led toxicology testing of its common commercial formulations, such as Roundup, because of research showing that when glyphosate is combined with other chemicals, as it is in Roundup and other glyphosate-based herbicides (GBH), the end product may be much more harmful than glyphosate alone. "A fresh and independent examination of GBH toxicity should be undertaken," and the government should "monitor GBH levels in people and in the food supply, none of which are occurring today," the scientists concluded.[25]

One of the commonly used co-formulants of concern in Roundup products has been a chemical called polyethoxylated tallow amine, or POEA, which works to help glyphosate penetrate the surface of plants. POEA is a type of "surfactant," an ingredient that helps the herbicide adhere to a plant instead of rolling off onto the soil. Monsanto has said POEA poses no danger, but researchers have determined that it actually can be up to 2,000 times more toxic to cells than glyphosate. Fish exposed to POEA in research studies have died, as have rats, even at low levels. Still, regulators have not focused assessments on these types of ingredients or how they interact with glyphosate. Some plaintiffs in the legal cases against Monsanto claim the company knew that robust safety studies were necessary for the combination of glyphosate with POEA in Roundup but skirted research that could have raised alarm bells.

Monsanto has been steadfast in denying any such dangers or allegations of lax research. Still, the company announced in 2016 that it would transition away from tallow amine in its products, saying the decision was due to "political debate," not any valid health concerns.[26] Monsanto's move came after European regulators started moving to ban POEA from glyphosate-based products.

Monsanto has long argued it has science on its side—that glyphosate has been proven safe and does not cause cancer and that there are no hidden dangers in Roundup's full package of ingredients. Regulators in the United States and numerous other countries have largely agreed with those safety assurances, and the company can point to a stack of research to back up its claims. More than 800 studies demonstrate glyphosate safety, the company says.[27] But critics are quick to point out that Monsanto's money helped fund a number of those studies, and some authors had consulting arrangements with the company. And it is notable, the critics say, that regulators have relied heavily on Monsanto-supplied studies when evaluating safety. Even research that might appear to be independent often is not. One of Monsanto's most touted studies,[28] which was published in 2000 and presented to the EPA and other regulatory bodies, appeared to be authored only by three scientists from outside the company. The paper appeared to be an independent review of research on glyphosate as well as POEA used in Roundup formulations and of the breakdown product aminomethylphosphonic acid (AMPA) and ultimately concluded that a thorough assessment proved there was nothing to fear. Not only was glyphosate not a carcinogen, but the researchers declared, "Roundup herbicide does not pose a health risk to humans." That research paper has been cited by hundreds of other publications. But the internal company documents that came to light in the Roundup lawsuits indicated that Monsanto scientists actually wrote that study. One Monsanto executive told colleagues in a February 2015 e-mail that they could "ghost-write" research materials and have certain independent scientists from outside the company "just edit & sign their names so to speak," just as they had done with the 2000 study.[29] The revelations outraged the plaintiffs. "Monsanto's ghostwriting has infected the scientific literature," plaintiffs' attorneys stated in court filings. "Monsanto is often the puppetmaster behind scientific articles that are positive for the company, as well as U.S. EPA deliberations and reports."[30]

Separate internal Monsanto records were almost equally unsettling, revealing company executives expressing dissatisfaction with a scientist who the company had asked to look at genotoxicity issues and who had come back with a list of concerns. If a substance is genotoxic, it can have a destructive effect on a cell's genetic material, its DNA, causing mutations. But internal e-mails from 1999 show company executives were unwilling to do the studies the scientist suggested needed to be done. Monsanto officials instead discussed a need to find someone else who might provide a more favorable view. The records also revealed discussions of seeking out "highly credible" scientists who could be paid for work to represent the safety of Monsanto products to regulators and fend off a "growing number of questionable genotoxicity publications."[31] The e-mails indicate that such scientists were recruited, and one key result was published research that shot down concerns about genotoxicity with glyphosate.[32]

After the internal communications became public, Monsanto argued that the records were taken out of context and did not accurately reflect company actions. The company insisted it did no ghostwriting, but rather only provided support and information to the authors of certain papers. But skeptics see the company documents as undermining the very foundation that regulators have used to vouch for Roundup's safety. Calls have come from the United States and Europe for regulators to throw out what appear to be tainted studies. "Monsanto tells us that Roundup is safe because scientists say it is safe. But apparently scientists sign their names, while Monsanto signs the checks. This calls into question multiple studies," said Kara Cook-Schultz of the United States Public Interest Research Group, based in Washington, DC.[33]

Monsanto insists that no other pesticide has been more extensively tested than glyphosate. Its safety has been proven in evaluations that span four decades, the company states. But while independent research that shows cause for alarm has been published for all to see, the company's own internal studies, which Monsanto says prove safety, are not available for public scrutiny because they are considered trade secrets. The ones that I've obtained make it clear that public scrutiny is not welcomed—each page is stamped with the warning "Contains Trade Secret or Otherwise Confidential Information of Monsanto Company." The EPA reinforces that message, warning anyone who obtains the studies that they are proprietary and cannot be posted or released for public viewing. Some of the research, which was presented years ago to the EPA, shows that test animals exposed to glyphosate did develop tumors or other irregularities, but those anomalies were judged by the researchers to be unrelated to the chemical exposure.

"Regulatory and scientific authorities worldwide have concluded that glyphosate when used according to label directions does not pose an unreasonable risk to human health, the environment or non-target animals and plants," Monsanto states.[34] But despite the company's assurances, over the past several years the body of publicly available research contradicting Monsanto has grown, making it hard to know just how dangerous this chemical agent could really be.

U.S. health officials have been trying for years to better understand not only glyphosate's impacts on farmers' health but also how the range of chemicals used in farming affects farmers and their families. Their primary research effort is a government-funded project known as the Agricultural Health Study (AHS). This massive collection of research data was launched in 1993 with funding from the National Cancer Institute and the National Institute of Environmental Health Sciences in collaboration with both the EPA and the National Institute for Occupational Safety and Health (NIOSH). The project looks at any connections between the many pesticides farmers spray on their fields and the higher rates of disease many farm communities seem to experience. The government has ample research suggesting higher rates of leukemia, myeloma, non-Hodgkin lymphoma, and cancers of the lip, stomach, skin, brain, and prostate for farmers when compared with people in more urban areas, but it hopes to use the AHS to determine more specifically just how significant the risks are and what may be done to lower those risks. More than 55,000 farmers and another 30,000-plus spouses are enrolled in the study, all from either Iowa or North Carolina, two top farming states chosen for the data gathering. From time to time, the participants get updates from the AHS researchers notifying them of new findings. They've been told, for instance, that a commonly used farm insecticide called diazinon is associated with an increased risk of ovarian cancer, and another widely used bug killer called malathion has been associated with an increased risk of thyroid cancer.

The study also has looked at the pesticide residues that invade farmers' homes. In a 2007 report, for instance, AHS researchers told the farm families that they had found residues of five different pesticides in carpet dust from their homes. The pesticide found at the highest levels of the five was glyphosate.

The study is still ongoing but has thus far found little or no connection between glyphosate and disease, including NHL. One 2005 AHS study of "glyphosate-exposed" farmers did suggest an "association" with multiple myeloma that researchers said should be followed up on.[35] Otherwise, the AHS data favor glyphosate safety, according to many scientists. But even that is the subject of some debate. Other scientists argue that government researchers looking at NHL cases have not yet followed farmers long enough to get a solid base of information on a disease that can take decades to develop. Several other studies looking at glyphosate and different types of cancer, such as brain and breast cancers, also show no connection.

For the average individual, reading through scientific research can be daunting, not to mention confusing. Different testing methodologies can lead to different results, and those results can often be interpreted in different ways. The scientific community relies not on one study, or two, but often on many dozens or hundreds of studies before it reaches a consensus. Many studies conclude not with definitive answers but with findings that add to a building body of knowledge.

Research about glyphosate's impacts has been drawing the attention of regulators, lawmakers, environmentalists, and consumers for years. In fact, the worrisome tumors found in rats and the other health issues researchers linked to glyphosate helped fuel efforts by U.S. consumer groups to force labeling of foods made with genetically engineered crops, because of the residues left after the crops are sprayed directly with glyphosate. But the general public did not take much notice of glyphosate until cancer experts with the World Health Organization's International Agency for Research on Cancer (IARC) stepped into the debate in March 2015.

~

The scientists who gathered in Lyon, France, on March 3, 2015, for a weeklong series of discussions about glyphosate did not expect the firestorm they were about to ignite. IARC does not aim to regulate substances but rather to identify things that can cause people to get cancer. The goal is to determine where hazards exist to inform individuals and to help regulators in efforts to protect public health. To that end, IARC pulls together different scientists from different specialties and different countries on a regular basis to look at various chemicals, drugs, mixtures, occupational exposures, and even lifestyles and personal habits. These IARC working groups have evaluated about 1,000 agents since 1971.

The group asked to evaluate glyphosate was made up of seventeen scientists from eleven countries. Along with glyphosate, they were also charged with analyzing research compiled on four other pesticides. Make no mistake: these were no amateurs. The scientists assembled were among the elite, roundly seen as independent experts, pulled from top institutions around the world. Frank Le Curieux, senior scientific officer at the European Chemicals Agency in Helsinki, Finland, and an expert in toxicology, was part of the team. So was French scientist Isabelle Baldi, who holds a doctorate in epidemiology, with a research specialty in environmental toxicology, and works as assistant professor in occupational epidemiology and public health at the University of Bordeaux. Another scientist on the team was Francesco Forastiere, head of occupational epidemiology at the Lazio Regional Health Service in Italy. Experts also came from Australia, New Zealand, Canada, the Netherlands, and Nicaragua. Five came from the United States, including Matthew Martin, a biologist and rising star with the EPA's National Center for Computational Toxicology, who has received numerous awards for his work with toxicity data.

And Aaron Blair, a scientist emeritus at the National Cancer Institute, served as chairman of the IARC team. Blair seemed the ideal candidate to lead the group—he had specialty knowledge in research that focused on evaluating cancer and other disease risks associated with agricultural exposures as well as chemicals in the workplace and the general environment. And he had a long career of accolades and appointments that acknowledged his expertise. After receiving his doctorate in genetics from North Carolina State University and a master of public health degree in epidemiology from the University of North Carolina, Blair joined the National Cancer Institute in 1976 and soon was named head of the Occupational Studies unit. He has received numerous awards over his career and has served on many national and international scientific review groups, including for the EPA. He has also authored more than 450 publications on occupational and environmental causes of cancer.

When he was named to lead IARC's working group, Blair had no reservations about taking on the glyphosate assignment. Industry players always take an interest when chemicals they profit from are up for IARC scrutiny, as they should. But Blair never expected that examining research would make him a target of Monsanto's ire. He would come to learn how wrong he was.

When the IARC team began its assessment, it was not charged with doing new research but rather with reviewing research already conducted, trying to determine how the various findings added up. IARC's process is typically tedious, to say the least. The assembling of relevant data generally begins several months before the working groups meet in person, and then the members generally spend long days in conference rooms analyzing data in subgroups, writing reports, and reviewing observations at the end of each day. The working group for glyphosate was no different. The members studiously analyzed older research as well as more recent studies, weighing the methods used, the consistency of results, and the levels of adherence to research standards. There were numerous animal studies to pore over, but fewer that looked directly at glyphosate's connections to health problems in humans.

For that latter category, the team gave particular consideration to major studies out of Sweden, Canada, and the United States.[36] The group determined that the best research showed a distinct association between non-Hodgkin lymphoma (NHL) and glyphosate. The team also noted that glyphosate was linked to multiple myeloma in three studies; however, the evidence for that disease was not as strong as the evidence tying glyphosate to NHL.

The team also evaluated several studies that showed animals developed rare kidney tumors and other health problems after exposure. The studies combined to provide "sufficient evidence" of glyphosate's carcinogenicity in laboratory animals, the IARC team found. On top of that, the IARC team concluded that there was strong evidence of genotoxicity and oxidative stress from glyphosate, including findings of chromosomal damage in the blood cells of people after glyphosate formulations were sprayed nearby.[37]

Overall, IARC concluded that there was "limited evidence" that glyphosate can cause cancer in humans and "sufficient evidence" that glyphosate can cause cancer in laboratory animals. The conclusion would have been for "sufficient" evidence of cancer problems for humans but for the Agricultural Health Study work done by the U.S. government that did not show definitive connections between cancer and glyphosate,

Forastiere, the working group member from Italy, told me. "The evidence was mixed on humans," he said.[38]

Under the classification system set up by IARC,[39] the group had five options—it could deem a substance "probably not" carcinogenic to humans; "not classifiable as to its carcinogenicity" to humans; "possibly" carcinogenic to humans; "probably carcinogenic" to humans; or the most definitive—"carcinogenic to humans." For a substance to be declared carcinogenic, the highest hazard level, there had to be "sufficient evidence" of cancer in humans or other similarly strong evidence. For the second rung, "probably carcinogenic," which was where glyphosate landed, scientists must find at least limited evidence of cancer ties in humans and sufficient evidence in animals. The team ultimately decided the weight of the evidence was not strong enough to put glyphosate in the most worrisome category, but it was more than enough to place it just below that. A Monsanto representative sat in on the deliberations and was given the opportunity to provide input but had no vote in the outcome.

"This chemical is a probable human carcinogen by any reasonable definition," said Christopher Portier, a toxicologist who was a nonvoting "invited specialist" to the IARC working group's work on glyphosate. "It is nonsense to say otherwise."[40] Portier was retired by that time, living in a remote village in Switzerland. But before his retirement, he had led the National Center for Environmental Health/Agency for Toxic Substances and Disease Registry at the Centers for Disease Control and Prevention (CDC), part of the U.S. Department of Health and Human Services. Prior to that role, Portier spent thirty-two years with the National Institute of Environmental Health Sciences (NIEHS), where he served as associate director, and director of the Environmental Toxicology Program, which has since merged into the institute's National Toxicology Program. His experience and high level of expertise had earned him credibility around the global scientific community. But critics of the glyphosate decision were quick to seize on the fact that in his retirement, Portier did some part-time consulting work with the Environmental Defense Fund, a nonprofit advocacy group. Portier's affiliation with the group, whose mission is "to preserve the natural systems on which all life depends," meant he was too biased to weigh in on glyphosate, industry advocates charged. Even though Portier did not vote on the IARC classification, his presence should be enough to discredit the findings, the industry players argued.

But Portier, Blair, Forastiere, and the other IARC scientists said they were more than comfortable with the validity of their work and proud of the thoroughness of what was a complicated undertaking. In a full report on the findings, the group underscored why the work matters. They cited research showing glyphosate can be found in soil, air, surface water, and groundwater and also cited studies showing glyphosate residues were easily found in food, including detections in 50 percent of cereal samples tested in Denmark and in six out of eight samples of tofu made from Brazilian soy. They also looked at data that showed glyphosate concentrations found in human urine, both in urban populations in Europe and in a rural population living near areas sprayed with glyphosate in Colombia.

"We knew that any determination from IARC would have been important because we knew the product was widespread and there was a lot of interest," Forastiere said.

~

What Forastiere and the other IARC scientists did not know was that Monsanto was tipped off to their decision on glyphosate before it was made public. Documents turned over in the court case show that the EPA gave Monsanto advance warning of the decision. So when IARC announced the results of its classification on March 20, 2015, Monsanto was ready with a counterassault. Monsanto's chairman, Hugh Grant, and other company officials asserted to reporters and investors that the classification by the elite group of scientists was "mischief" based on "junk science" and politically motivated. The company issued a statement reaffirming that "glyphosate and glyphosate-based herbicides are among the most thoroughly tested and evaluated pesticide products in the world. Their 40-year history of safe use is supported by one of the most extensive worldwide human health, crop residue and environmental databases ever compiled on any pesticide."[41] The company also angrily demanded a retraction from IARC. And Monsanto wasted no time in calling on the EPA to defend glyphosate against the cancer claims. IARC's announcement was made on a Friday, and by the following Monday morning, Monsanto's Dan Jenkins, who led the company's U.S. regulatory affairs work at that time, was e-mailing and calling contacts at the EPA, providing the agency with "talking points" and urging the agency to "correct mistakes or absences of fact with respect to its record on glyphosate . . . as it relates to carcinogenicity."[42]

Monsanto's Philip Miller, vice president for global regulatory affairs, penned a letter to Margaret Chan, director-general of the World Health Organization (WHO), complaining that IARC "purposefully chose to disregard dozens of studies" supporting the safety of glyphosate. Miller said the company was "anxious" to address the issue. "Safety is our number one priority, and we know that IARC's conclusions will likely cause a great deal of concern with growers and consumers alike," Miller wrote.[43]

IARC's director, Christopher Wild, wrote back affirming the agency's support for the team's classification of glyphosate as a probable human carcinogen, calling the finding the result of a "comprehensive review of the latest available scientific evidence."[44]

CropLife International, an agrochemical industry association, also stepped into the fray, sending a series of letters to IARC and WHO expressing concerns and asking for a "clarification," saying IARC's findings "have undermined our work with regulators."[45]

The decision by IARC could not have come at a worse time for Monsanto. In the spring of 2015, the EPA was wrapping up a years-long reregistration assessment of glyphosate that was supposed to look at potential evolving risks and see if there was any reason to limit the use of glyphosate. Before IARC's announcement, glyphosate was slated for a green light; the new registration report was nearly completed and was planned for release to the public later in 2015. Monsanto was also working to roll out a new herbicide that combined glyphosate with another weed-killing chemical called dicamba, along with new herbicide-tolerant crops to go with it. As well, the company was undergoing a similar reregistration assessment of glyphosate in Europe. With all that at stake, the IARC report was so potentially damning that Monsanto simply could not let it stand.

Internal company documents show that within two months of IARC's classification, Monsanto was laying out a plan to spend potentially upward of $200,000 to provide a powerful counterpunch aimed at discrediting the IARC scientists and their work. The IARC classification was a "severe stigma" that had to be addressed, according to an internal report that laid out a series of proposals for "scientific projects" to show glyphosate's safety. For one project looking at animal test data, the "majority of the writing can be done by Monsanto" to keep costs down, even though the project would have "external authors." Another, broader project called for assembling a panel of "credible scientists" to publish a "comprehensive evaluation" of glyphosate's cancer-causing potential. Again, Monsanto hoped to do much of the writing to keep costs down but pegged the costs at $200,000 to $250,000.[46] Monsanto tried to keep the document laying out those details confidential, but it became public as part of the Roundup litigation.

Monsanto's panel of scientists was formed in July 2015, and in December the researchers reported—perhaps not surprisingly—that IARC was flat out wrong in classifying glyphosate the way it had. The panel said the IARC scientists had incorrectly weighted or ignored data and that there was no evidence of "human carcinogenesis." Ten of the sixteen scientists on that panel had worked as consultants for Monsanto in the past, and two more were former Monsanto employees. But Monsanto insisted publicly that the report was "independent" and maintained that it was more valid than the work of the IARC scientists.[47] The team of sixteen scientists then went on to publish their findings of glyphosate safety in a scientific journal called *Critical Reviews in Toxicology.* Some unsuspecting journalists reported on the panel's findings as though they were in fact independent and equal in weight to the IARC findings that they contradicted.

Despite Monsanto's efforts, concerns over the IARC classification were not quelled. Lawmakers and regulators in many countries had already taken notice of the red flags being waved around glyphosate before IARC's news and were moving to limit use of the chemical. After the cancer classification, those moves intensified. Consumer protection officials in Germany called for a European Union–wide ban on glyphosate use by individuals; France restricted glyphosate sales to the public; Italy banned the use of glyphosate in public places and those frequented by children and the elderly; Colombia temporarily suspended the use of glyphosate to spray coca plants; Sri Lanka banned the importation of glyphosate; and—in an action that specifically rankled Monsanto—California said it would add glyphosate to a list of chemicals known to cause cancer.

Monsanto fired back against California's action, suing state environmental regulators to try to block them from putting glyphosate on the list.[48] Monsanto argued the move would cost the company sales and force it to provide a warning on its products—something Monsanto said would violate its right to free speech. A judge in the case ruled against Monsanto, allowing the state to require warnings about Roundup. In its lawsuit, Monsanto took the opportunity to assail the IARC scientists again, characterizing the group as an "unelected, undemocratic, unaccountable, and foreign body."

The uproar over their classification and the attacks on their credibility caught the IARC scientists off guard. "We were not expecting this strong reaction and what happened," Forastiere recalled. "We were doing our job. I understood there were other issues . . . economic consequences. But none of us had a political agenda. We are scientists."[49] Forastiere retreated and shunned hundreds of interview requests from media around the world. He and the other scientists who were not based in the United States were able to insulate themselves from the criticism a bit more easily than was Blair, who had to return home to U.S. soil, Monsanto's home base. Monsanto soon subpoenaed Blair's e-mails and other documents to try to discredit the IARC working group's findings.

Throughout the uproar, the EPA provided much-needed aid to Monsanto, intentionally or not. Two months after the IARC bombshell, the EPA said it had reviewed thirty-two studies that specifically analyzed whether or not glyphosate might be an endocrine disruptor, which if true would mean glyphosate indeed could cause cancer, along with infertility, diabetes, or other problems. But the EPA said there was nothing to fear, for the studies proved glyphosate's safety. What the EPA did not say was that twenty-seven of the thirty-two studies were either conducted by or funded by Monsanto or its industry allies. Only five of the studies considered by the EPA were independent, and three of those five did in fact find that the chemical could pose a threat. Even many of the industry's own studies had findings that could suggest exposure to glyphosate was dangerous, but when the animals exposed to glyphosate suffered health problems or died, the scientists for these industry-backed studies dismissed the results as not valid.[50]

And, in what would become a highly controversial move, the EPA's own cancer experts, the Cancer Assessment Review Committee (CARC), responded to IARC's classification with a report that purported to re-evaluate the issue. And again, the agency found no cause for alarm, determining that the best literature showed glyphosate was "not likely" to cause cancer. The group did hedge its bets with respect to non-Hodgkin lymphoma, however, citing "conflicting evidence for the association between glyphosate exposure and NHL." Because of that lack of clarity surrounding NHL, the group said this: "While epidemiologic literature to date does not support a direct causal association, the CARC recommends that the literature should continue to be monitored for studies related to glyphosate and risk of NHL."[51]

The EPA's Office of Research and Development (ORD), the scientific research arm of the EPA, reviewed the agency's glyphosate cancer analysis internally and found it flawed in many ways, lacking support for the finding of "not likely" to cause cancer. The ORD said the agency had not followed its own guidelines in coming to its conclusion. The EPA did not budge, however, sticking with its defense of glyphosate's safety.[52]

What observers did not know at the time, but learned later as the company's internal documents were unsealed in the Roundup litigation, is that Monsanto had an especially helpful and well-placed ally within the EPA. A longtime agency scientist named Jesudoss "Jess" Rowland was in close communication with Monsanto regarding glyphosate's review and was seen by the company as someone who could be especially "useful" in defending glyphosate. Rowland served at the time as the deputy division director within the Health Effects Division of the EPA's Office of Pesticide Programs, managing the work of scientists who assessed human health effects of exposures to pesticides like glyphosate. And, importantly, he chaired the EPA's Cancer Assessment Review Committee (CARC), which issued the report that contradicted IARC's findings.

Rowland had a long history of taking a favorable position on Monsanto's glyphosate—in 1998, Rowland and the hazard identification assessment review committee where he served as executive secretary recommended that the EPA drop the extra safety margin designed to protect children in the agency's reevaluation of what constituted a safe dose of glyphosate.[53] So it is not surprising that Monsanto turned to him after the IARC decision.

E-mails obtained from the EPA through the Freedom of Information Act (FOIA) show that there were telephone communications between a Monsanto executive and Rowland about Monsanto's desire for the EPA to help counter IARC. Details of what the two may have said to each other are unknown. But an internal Monsanto document says that Rowland told Monsanto at one point that he would try to kill an additional review of glyphosate planned by the Agency for Toxic Substances and Disease Registry, a unit of the U.S. Department of Health and Human Services. And indeed, as of this writing, no such review has occurred.[54]

More help from inside the EPA was seen in an odd event in the spring of 2016. Rowland's CARC report, which was so favorable to Monsanto, was not supposed to be made public for many more months, as it was intended to inform a broader EPA report still under way. But on Friday, April 29, the CARC report mysteriously appeared on the EPA's website. Monsanto immediately copied the report and then touted it on the company website. The report remained on the EPA's website for three days before the EPA pulled it down and issued a public statement saying it was "inadvertently" posted. It may have been only three days, but the documents still got wide play in global news outlets as Monsanto pointed to helpful EPA language in the report such as this: "The epidemiological evidence at this time does not support a causal relationship between glyphosate exposure and solid tumors. There is also no evidence to support a causal relationship between glyphosate exposure and the following non-solid tumors: leukemia, multiple myeloma, or Hodgkin lymphoma. The epidemiological evidence at this time is inconclusive for a causal or clear associative relationship between gly-phosate and NHL."[55]

The report gave Monsanto fresh ammunition as it battled to quell the mounting number of lawsuits brought by people who said Roundup gave them or family members cancer. The company even took a copy of the report to a key May 3 court hearing to help defend itself against the lawsuits.

The temporary publication of the helpful report also came, coincidentally or not, shortly before a key European vote on whether or not to reauthorize glyphosate in the European Union, which was scheduled for May 2016. The vote ultimately was postponed.

Skeptics smelled a rat, but the EPA refused to answer questions about the CARC report and refused to comply with FOIA requests seeking agency documents that might explain the fiasco. Rowland left his twenty-six-year career at the EPA shortly after the leak and sequestered himself, ducking questions from me and other reporters. Interestingly enough, Monsanto knew in advance Rowland was ready to leave the agency. Jenkins, the company's regulatory affairs leader, told his colleagues as much in a September 2015 e-mail, saying, "Jess will be retiring from EPA in ~5–6 mos and could be useful as we move forward with ongoing glyphosate defense."[56]

The conversations revealed in the documents show nothing less than "a concerted effort by Monsanto and the OPP, Jess Rowland, and his CARC committee, to 'kill' the glyphosate/lymphoma issue for the company," the plaintiffs' attorneys stated in a court filing. "The documentary evidence strongly suggests that Mr. Rowland's primary goal was to serve the interests of Monsanto."[57]

Rowland was later forced by the federal judge overseeing the Roundup cancer litigation to sit for a deposition and acknowledged, only after a specific order from the judge, that after he left the EPA he started doing some consulting work for chemical industry interests, including two that "are among Monsanto's closest associates," court filings submitted by plaintiffs' attorneys stated.[58] Rowland refused to provide details about how much he was being paid or the details of how and when he got the jobs, and the judge in the case declined to allow Rowland to be pressed further.

The CARC report authored by Rowland was certainly key for Monsanto, but the EPA's defense of glyphosate didn't stop there. In September 2016, the agency published a 227-page report stating definitively that its best experts had determined glyphosate was "not likely" to cause cancer in humans.[59] Agency officials said their findings were based in part on unpublished studies submitted by Monsanto and other industry players. That differed from the work of the IARC group, which had focused on peer-reviewed, published studies.

Notably, Martin, the EPA research biologist who was part of the IARC working group that declared glyphosate probably cancer-causing, was not included on the EPA's own team that evaluated glyphosate for cancer links.

To strengthen its glyphosate safety determination, the agency announced it would seek input from independent experts on the matter. When dealing with tricky scientific issues involving chemical research, the EPA often sets up what it calls a Scientific Advisory Panel (SAP), which it stacks with the best and brightest minds it can find in toxicology, epidemiology, microbiology, and other relevant disciplines. The meetings are open to the public, offering a glimpse into the often dry—but important—discourse that goes into classifying chemical risk. For glyphosate, the EPA did the same, signing up leading research specialists from around the United States to come together and advise the agency on its view that glyphosate was unlikely to be carcinogenic to people. The EPA specifically said it would be good to have a careful review of existing epidemiologic data, given the IARC determination.

Monsanto did not want the outside scientists brought in, did not want the SAP on glyphosate to be held. Such a panel of independent experts could "create legal vulnerabilities," an internal Monsanto document stated.[60] Publicly, Monsanto called the SAP "an unnecessary use of resources."[61] But, to its credit, the EPA refused to back away from the plan, setting the four-day meetings for mid-October 2016.

Still, even this seemingly public-minded move by the EPA would become an example of the power of industry influence. When it became clear that the EPA would go ahead with the gathering of scientific experts, industry executives made their ire known. The U.S. trade group CropLife America, which is funded by Monsanto and other makers of agrochemicals, complained in writing to the EPA that the meetings were a waste of taxpayers' time and said it had "significant concerns" about the prospects of a public meeting on the issue.[62]

CropLife argued that if the meetings were to be held, at least one of the independent scientists chosen to help advise the EPA was not suitable.[63] CropLife specifically called for the EPA to remove Peter Infante, an expert in epidemiology, from the panel.

The demand was a bold one: Infante was world-renowned after spending twenty-four years with the U.S. Department of Labor's Occupational Safety and Health Administration, helping to determine cancer risks to workers during the development of standards for toxic substances including asbestos, arsenic, benzene, and formaldehyde. His résumé also included a stint at the National Institute for Occupational Safety and Health, where he conducted epidemiological studies related to carcinogens, and he had served as an expert consultant in epidemiology for several world bodies, including IARC and the World Trade Organization (WTO). In 1999, Infante was chosen as one of four epidemiologists to advise the WTO during its deliberations on the European Union's ban of chrysotile asbestos. But CropLife told the EPA that the chemical industry players it represented feared Infante would disregard industry-funded studies in favor of independent research. They said he had showed bias in the past against the industry and had testified in a past court case against Monsanto. He had to go, CropLife said.

The EPA caved. Two days after the agency received the October 12, 2016, CropLife letter asking for Infante's ouster, the EPA said it was halting the meetings that were to have run from October 18 to October 21. The EPA refused to acknowledge that the move was due to industry arm-twisting and said the change was due to scheduling conflicts. It also said it needed to find additional epidemiology expertise.[64] Oddly, no one told Infante he was off the panel. Weeks went by in which Infante continued to receive SAP documents from the EPA and was led to believe he was still to be part of the scientific team. But when the EPA finally announced in November that it was rescheduling the meetings for December, Infante's name was missing from the SAP roster of experts. Infante was confused; he had not been notified of his exclusion until the day before the rescheduled dates were announced. The appearance of industry influence was obvious, but the agency did its best to deflect publicity around Infante's dismissal, hinting that he had simply become "unavailable" to serve on the panel and refusing to discuss the decision in detail with reporters.

Infante, who lives in the Virginia suburbs within a short drive of the EPA offices, was outraged at the agency's actions. He had served as an expert on an unrelated scientific panel only a year prior for the EPA without issue. "Can you think of one other chemical that has more impact—economic and other—than glyphosate? That's why I'm not on the panel. Monsanto didn't want me on there and they figured out a way to get me off," he said.

Monsanto and others in the agrochemical industry elite often act like "bullies," according to Infante. "If scientists have a lot of integrity, then they try to destroy them," he said. "We live in a society of risks, and in a free society a person should be able to make an informed choice based on knowledge of the risks. But the industry tries to obscure the knowledge. How can the public even hope to get independent scientific findings?"[65]

When the EPA held the SAP meetings in mid-December 2016, Infante showed up anyway. Before being removed from the panel, he had spent countless hours going through the research, and he wanted to make sure his observations were heard. He asked the EPA to allow him to speak during the public comments portion of the meeting and was told he could have ten minutes. He dressed conservatively for the occasion, in a dark suit and shirt, but added a splashy bright orange and silver tie. He made no mention of his treatment by the EPA when delivering his public remarks and focused only on what he said were significant findings in the epidemiology data. Looking every bit the professor with his manicured gray goatee, wire-rimmed glasses, and a somewhat unruly mound of thinning curls atop his head, Infante commanded rapt attention from the other scientists as he conveyed his analysis. His conclusion, he told the other panel members, was "impressive evidence" of ties between NHL and glyphosate. He told the group that the epidemiological data showed that glyphosate should be considered a likely human carcinogen.

"There is clearly the evidence for the risk of non-Hodgkin lymphoma related to glyphosate exposure," Infante said. "Is it conclusive? No, I don't think so. But I think that EPA is concluding that there is no evidence. And that's exactly wrong."[66]

Several members of the Scientific Advisory Panel had their own concerns about the EPA's dismissive view of some of the data showing links to cancer, and they said as much during the public meetings. Some scientists said they were concerned that the EPA was violating its own guidelines in discounting data from various studies that show positive associations between glyphosate and cancer. And some questioned why the EPA excluded some data that showed statistical significance and wrote off some of the positive findings to mere chance. Monique Perron, a scientist in the Health Effects Division of the EPA's Office of Pesticide Programs, tried to explain away the concerns, telling the assembled scientists that "professional judgment" played a role in looking at the "weight of evidence" from various studies.

Still, panel member Lianne Sheppard, assistant chair in the Department of Environmental and Occupational Health Sciences at the University of Washington School of Public Health, said there was enough epidemiological evidence linking glyphosate to NHL to support a "suggestive" causal connection. Individually, the studies may not contain strong evidence of a connection between glyphosate exposure and NHL, but when looked at together, they do, she said. "Clearly, it's suggestive to me, and it's the most appropriate public health conclusion to reach," she said.

Panelist Kenneth Portier, a statistician with the American Cancer Society and brother to IARC advisor Christopher Portier, noted the split between the scientists on how to weigh the research. "Rarely does a panel disagree as much as this one," Portier said.[67]

Aside from the discussions of the science, some onlookers questioned whether the EPA gave nonindustry experts fair time. During what the EPA deemed the "public comments" part of the agenda, Monsanto representatives were granted roughly three and one-half hours to argue their case for glyphosate safety, and several other agrochemical industry players were allowed lengthy presentations as well. In comparison, most critics of glyphosate had comment periods that ranged from five to fifteen minutes. EPA spokesman Steven Knott said that assignments of speaking allotments were based on how much time commentators asked for, but some glyphosate opponents said they were told they could not have more than a few minutes.

Monsanto used its time to present a defense of glyphosate's value to agriculture, to offer detailed explanations for why IARC's analysis was flawed, and to explain why the company believed that a host of data points found in various studies should be discounted or are not relevant. Company representatives also argued that glyphosate residues found in numerous urine tests were nothing to worry about and actually helped show that the chemical does not bioaccumulate in the human body. They also said reports of glyphosate residues found in human breast milk were "implausible."

Any doubts the EPA or its scientific advisors might have had about how much attention the public was paying to the meetings disappeared as several members of consumer and environmental groups showed up to implore the EPA to restrict or ban the chemical. Kathy Blum, a "concerned mother" from Leesburg, Virginia, and a member of the Moms Across America group, was one of the first to take the microphone, her voice rising as she made her plea. "Glyphosate is everywhere. It's in our air, our water, our soil, our food, our beverages, it's in mothers' breast milk," she told the panel. "Children are exposed to glyphosate in many areas, playgrounds, parks, ballfields, and their own backyards. Glyphosate has been found in tap water, our children's urine. Any amount of glyphosate is unacceptable. By allowing glyphosate-based herbicides to be sprayed on our food and feed crops you are allowing America to be poisoned through our food and water. All of us are guinea pigs in this horrendous toxic experiment. You have an opportunity now to stop this. Our lives depend on it."

A poignant moment also came when Alexis Baden-Mayer, a lawyer with the Organic Consumers Association, read aloud letters to the EPA written by people blaming Roundup for lymphomas that struck them or their family members. One letter was written by Vicky Laybourne, whose husband, Paul, died of central nervous system lymphoma after years of exposure to Roundup. Vicky and Paul had been married for forty-three years and were happily settling into semiretirement when Paul became sick. Vicky, who lives in Smithville, Missouri, couldn't attend the EPA meetings in person, but she wanted the EPA to know what her family went through when the cancer was found in Paul's brain and he died in September 2012. "I wasn't aware how widespread this was," she told me. "These companies need to be held accountable."[68]

The EPA meetings even drew theatrics as a New York–based activist known as the Reverend Billy Talen, who leads a group of self-proclaimed "earth-loving urban activists," took his turn at the microphone. Accompanied by fellow activist Robin Laverne Wilson, who goes by the moniker Dragonfly, Talen told the EPA and scientific advisors that his group had created a national map of parks and playgrounds where glyphosate is used to aid parents who want to avoid exposure to the chemical. "There is a political cloud hanging over this room, this proceeding," he said. Clad in a minister's dark robe and white collar, Talen told the EPA and scientists that they should "pull the curtain back" and expose the political pressure that Monsanto applies to keep glyphosate on the market. "We ask you to free yourself from this tremendous prejudice that has kept this toxin in so many of our homes, in our bodies, in our food, in our air." When Talen and his group exhausted their allotted five minutes, they launched into song, repeating a solemn, hymnlike refrain: "Monsanto is the devil. No glyphosate."

When the meeting was over, panel members wrote a final report to the EPA that said they could not fully agree with the EPA's view of glyphosate safety. While some agreed that evidence of carcinogenicity was lacking, other panel members felt the research did "suggest a potential for glyphosate to affect cancer incidence." And the group agreed with many critics who said that the EPA was improperly discounting the findings of some studies. "Many of the arguments put forth" by the EPA as supporting glyphosate safety "are not persuasive," panel members concluded.[69] As of this writing, however, the EPA has done nothing to rein in the use of glyphosate, and its final risk assessment—initially due out in 2015—is still pending.

The EPA's actions are particularly vexing to many who believe the agency is relying on outdated, industry-funded research and undue industry guidance in making its determinations. And they fear the public is suffering for it.

"Glyphosate is a very effective herbicide . . . but it should be extremely restricted," said Thierry Vrain, a soil biologist and genetic scientist who spent thirty years working for Canada's national agricultural department. "The stupidity of having it in the crops is madness and the level of exposure to people is unacceptable. The residues in the food are probably responsible for a lot more damage to humans than anything else."

Vrain did not come easily to his criticism. In fact, he was a long-time defender of technological advances in agriculture. During graduate school in North Carolina in the 1970s, Vrain learned all about the wide range of pests and pathogens that can lay ruin to a critical crop, so he was particularly enthusiastic when genetically engineered crops were introduced that could resist harmful pests, and he held faith that the biotech companies would do as they promised and develop disease-resistant crops as well. All he really knew about the Roundup herbicide that so many farmers were using with these GMOs and other crops was that "Roundup was supposed to be the best thing on earth," Vrain recalls. "'It was wonderful,' everyone said."[70]

When Vrain retired from the agriculture department in June 2003, he had so much time on his hands that he took up gardening and started learning more about organic agriculture. He began to examine how the prevalent use of Roundup might be more perilous than many people suspected. Vrain pored over scientific journals and obscure studies examining glyphosate, and what he found disturbed him so much that he pushed aside the relaxation of retirement to take on an activist's role, working to convince Canadian and U.S. regulators of what he sees as serious human and environmental hazards.

Regulators have simply become too entwined with corporate interests to be objective about the high-dollar products pushed by the powerful chemical industry, Vrain believes. "Everybody can be influenced," he said. "Corporations have a lot of money, and they know how to work the system."[71]

CHAPTER 6

Spinning the Science

For every scientist who raises a concern about a product, there seems to be a corporation to contradict him (or her). We've seen this happen again and again. Tobacco industry executives famously hid research done by their own scientists that showed the hazards of cigarettes, and they misled lawmakers and regulators about the addictive properties of nicotine. Many other corporate powers, including those in the agrochemical industry, have long histories of defending themselves against claims that they covered up the dangers of injury from asbestos, polychlorinated biphenyls (PCBs), Agent Orange, or other chemicals.

DuPont has spent the past several years in an ongoing battle against more than 3,000 lawsuits alleging the company knew that a chemical called perfluorooctanoic acid, commonly known as PFOA, could cause disease but hid that knowledge for decades even as its PFOA contaminated West Virginia water supplies.[1] And Dow AgroSciences spent years fighting mightily to stop the U.S. Environmental Protection Agency (EPA) from banning an insecticide tied to brain damage in children.

Like any corporation, Monsanto Company does not shy away from zealously using its money, power, and political sway to promote its products and defend them against criticism. That is to be expected. But with

Monsanto and its allies in the agrochemical industry, the propaganda playbook has many different chapters—and some are intentionally hard to read.

A common tactic is to funnel industry messaging through individuals who appear to be independent of industry and who carry a gloss of expertise and acclaim that gives them credibility with consumers, lawmakers, and regulators. These "experts" appear unaffiliated with industry and thus unbiased. What the public doesn't know is that behind the scenes, corporations are often funding and collaborating closely with these very same professors and other professionals who tout propaganda that serves industry interests. It's all part of a strategy of spin that has been used by the tobacco industry, the soft drink industry, pharmaceuticals, and, of course, agriculture.

These closeted collaborations make it difficult for consumers to know whom to trust and what to believe. And the rule appears to be "The less transparent, the better." Several examples have come to light only because of records obtained through Freedom of Information Act (FOIA) requests and investigations by journalists and consumer and environmental groups. What the records clearly show is a roster of U.S. academics—people employed by taxpayer-funded institutions—quietly working with Monsanto, other agrochemical companies, and public relations experts to tout the benefits of company products, to counter anything that points to problems with glyphosate or glyphosate-tolerant crops, and to cripple unfavorable legislation or regulation. The ties to the industry are typically not disclosed as these people sell the story the corporations want told.

One example of the hidden corporate hand at work dates back to 2013, when Monsanto wanted to procure "policy briefs" supportive of the company's interests that appeared to be unaffiliated with the company. The plan was laid out by Monsanto's chief of global scientific affairs, Eric Sachs, in an e-mail to nine prominent academics, including a professor at the prestigious Harvard Kennedy School. Sachs told the professors he hoped each would help with an initiative to promote the "safety and benefits" of genetically modified organisms (GMOs), and he assigned each a topic and background materials. Harvard professor Calestous Juma was asked to write an article laying out the "consequences of rejecting GM crops." Each brief "should be about 4–6 pages in length and include key themes and messages related to the specific topic, recommendations, and a call to action" aimed at a broad audience that included policy makers and regulators, Sachs told the professors.

"The key to success is participation by all of you—recognized experts and leaders with the knowledge, reputation and communication experience needed to communicate authoritatively to the target groups. You represent an elite group whose credibility will be strengthened by working together. . . . You are the best possible messengers," Sachs wrote.[2]

Sachs told the group that an organization called the American Council on Science and Health would run the project in partnership with a public relations consulting group. The plan was for the two organizations to coordinate the publishing and promotion of the articles, setting up speaking engagements, webinars, and other events. Sachs said he was aware that the professors' reputations "must be protected" and that "Monsanto wants the authors to communicate freely without involvement by Monsanto." By December 2014, the articles Monsanto had asked for were circulating, though without any mention that they came at Monsanto's behest.[3] Juma's article hewed closely to Monsanto's suggestions. The connections came to light only when the e-mail communications were obtained through FOIA requests from the consumer advocacy group U.S. Right to Know and reported by several news outlets. For his part, Juma told the *Boston Globe* that he may have used "bad judgment" but didn't intend to hide Monsanto's ties. He received no money for the work and was true to his own views, he said.[4]

Another prime example of hidden alliances has come to be known as the "Séralini affair." Gilles-Eric Séralini was a professor of molecular biology at the University of Caen Normandy when he published a study in September 2012 in a scientific journal called *Food and Chemical Toxicology* (FCT) about the effects of Roundup herbicide and Roundup Ready corn on 200 rats. Publication in a journal such as FCT requires a lengthy process in which experts unrelated to the study review it and can ask questions and seek revisions before it is published. This peer review process is meant to curb publication of flawed research.

Séralini had spent two years and more than $3 million working with seven other scientists to study how the genetically modified corn and the herbicide impacted the animals' health. At the time, Séralini was also president of a scientific advisory board that worked with a group opposed to GMOs. He believed there were potential problems with GMOs and Roundup that had not yet been uncovered by the scientific research that was largely funded by the chemical industry. Séralini and his team had seen troubling results in previous studies, including evidence that Roundup herbicides containing POEA along with glyphosate were much more harmful than glyphosate alone, causing cell damage at levels expected to be found in food.[5]

Groups of rats were evaluated by the Séralini team in the 2012 study. The rats were divided into males and females. Some were fed genetically engineered corn; others consumed corn sprayed in the field with Roundup; and others were given Roundup in drinking water in different doses, with the lowest corresponding to levels found in some tap water. The intermediate dose was set at the maximum level permitted in the United States in animal feed, and the highest dose was correlated to half the strength of Roundup as used in agriculture. Control group rats were fed a diet containing non–genetically engineered corn and plain drinking water.

The Séralini study results were alarming. Treated rats had much higher death rates than the control group animals, and the exposed rats demonstrated an "unexpected increase in tumor incidence," especially mammary tumors in female rats, along with damage to the animals' livers and kidneys. The scientists said both the GMO corn and Roundup contributed to the health problems that developed in the experimental animals, and they said they found "unexpected low dose toxicity from Roundup" at levels 10,000 times lower than those permitted in drinking water in the United States.[6] The study results "clearly indicate that lower levels of complete agricultural G [glyphosate] herbicide formulations, at concentrations well below officially set safety limits, can induce severe hormone-dependent mammary, hepatic, and kidney disturbances," the study authors concluded.[7] Séralini said his research gave credence to fears that Roundup contains ingredients more toxic than glyphosate and that Roundup formulations should be considered endocrine disruptors.

News outlets around the world published stories about the study findings, and regulators in many countries were understandably rattled. France's prime minister at the time, Jean-Marc Ayrault, said that the country would consider a ban on GMO corn sprayed with glyphosate, and the European Commission said it would seek a review by the European Food Safety Authority. Russia temporarily suspended importing glyphosate-tolerant corn, and Kenya actually moved to ban all GMO crops, most of which were sprayed directly with glyphosate.

The announcement of the study results came at a particularly bad time for Monsanto, just two months before California residents were slated to vote on whether or not to require labeling of foods made with GMOs, an issue Monsanto adamantly opposed. Glyphosate residue on foods was one of the concerns that drove the labeling efforts, not just in California but in several other states as well, so any bad news about glyphosate's impacts on health was a big problem. Just as they had done with other negative research reports and not unlike the attack they would later launch against the International Agency for Research on Cancer (IARC), Monsanto and associated industry players railed against the Séralini study, telling journalists it was fatally flawed in many ways. The European Federation of Biotechnology industry association, which counts Monsanto and other agribusiness firms among its members, called for the paper to be retracted, saying it reflected a "dangerous failure of the peer-review system." Other organizations and ultimately regulatory bodies weighed in, mimicking Monsanto's claims that the research was flawed and not to be believed. California voters narrowly rejected the mandatory GMO labeling bill as the attacks on Séralini continued for well over a year and scientists around the world debated the perceived merits and shortcomings of the Séralini work.

About 130 scientists, scholars, and activists took Séralini's side, weighing in with support in an open letter published in *Independent Science News*. The group noted the industry pressure on scientists whose findings were unfavorable and said the backlash against Séralini's study raised "the profile of fundamental challenges faced by science in a world increasingly dominated by corporate influence."[8]

And then Richard Goodman stepped in. Goodman, a trim, bookish-looking man who favored a neatly kept moustache and held a doctorate in dairy science, worked for Monsanto from 1997 to 2004. But by the fall of 2012, when the Séralini study was published, Goodman was working at the University of Nebraska–Lincoln.

Records would reveal that despite his work at the public university, Goodman was still tightly entwined with Monsanto, relying on funding from the company and other agrochemical interests to run a food allergy research program at the University of Nebraska. In that role, he was happily touting the safety of agricultural biotechnology, training scientists from other countries in how to evaluate the safety of GMO crops that are sprayed with glyphosate, and issuing reports about how GMO crops, engineered to be sprayed with glyphosate or to repel pests, were not likely to trigger allergic reactions in people. And though Goodman's job description listed him as a faculty member of the university's

Department of Food Science and Technology, it was the funding from Monsanto and other agrochemical and seed companies, such as Bayer, DuPont, and Syngenta, that kept Goodman afloat. A look at the sponsorship agreement for the allergen database for 2013 showed that each of six sponsoring companies was to pay roughly $51,000 for a total budget of $308,154 for that year. Goodman was also collaborating with Monsanto on efforts to turn back mandatory GMO labeling efforts and mitigate GMO safety concerns and was offered "media training" by the agrobusinesses. Records would reveal that roughly half of Goodman's income came through industry funding.

When the Séralini study broke, Goodman was quickly in contact with Monsanto officials and eager to help in the response. Documents, again obtained by U.S. Right to Know, show that on the day the Séralini study was published—September 19, 2012—Goodman was e-mailing Monsanto toxicologist Bruce Hammond shortly before 10 a.m., asking for "talking points, or bullet analysis" that Goodman could use in discussing the study.[9]

By November, Goodman was doing much more: he was acting as associate editor of the FCT scientific journal—the very one that had just published the Séralini study and from which Monsanto was seeking a retraction. Goodman was placed in a role overseeing GMO-related research reports. It's not clear if Monsanto had a hand in getting Goodman appointed, but e-mails do show a direct connection between Monsanto's Hammond, Goodman, and FCT's editor-in-chief, A. Wallace Hayes. Shortly after Goodman was named associate editor, Hayes told Hammond that he and Goodman were aware of the criticism of the Séralini paper and wanted Hammond and other critics to act as reviewers for the journal.[10] Around the same time Goodman was signing on to FCT, he was also worrying about whether the industry money would keep flowing. In e-mails, he expressed concern about protecting his income stream as a "soft-money professor."[11]

In late 2013, after Goodman had been on the journal's editorial team for roughly a year, FCT abruptly retracted the Séralini study, saying it had decided the data were inconclusive and the conclusions unreliable. Critics were quick to link the retraction to Goodman, but he denied any involvement. Séralini saw a clear connection, however. In a statement defending his work, he declared the retraction the result of "pressure from the GMO and agrochemical industry to force acceptance of GMOs and Roundup." Goodman's appointment to the editorial team was a "most flagrant illustration" of agrobusiness's influence and underscored how industry's tight hold on what was considered acceptable science "puts public health at risk," he said.[12]

"This episode illustrated the vulnerable position of dependent 'science' and the economic and political forces that move to defend Roundup and Roundup-contaminated crops," Séralini said.[13] The Séralini study was republished in another journal, *Environmental Sciences Europe*, in June 2014. Still, the heavy industry criticism left Séralini's credibility deeply scarred.

Goodman's affiliation with Monsanto was underscored by communications related to a second study, the Sri Lanka work that tied glyphosate to kidney disease.[14] E-mails obtained show Goodman asked Monsanto's Food Safety Scientific Affairs lead, John Vicini, in October 2014 for help evaluating what he called an "anti-paper." Goodman said he needed someone at Monsanto to provide him with some "sound scientific arguments" for how to view the study's findings.[15] Monsanto actively campaigned to discredit the study, saying there was no evidence whatsoever that glyphosate contributes to kidney failure in humans or animals.

Another professor with close, but largely hidden, ties to Monsanto (who also called for a retraction of the Séralini study) is former University of Illinois food science professor Bruce Chassy. Prior to his retirement in 2012, Chassy touted a stellar academic reputation and decades of experience earned at the public university and as a researcher at the

National Institutes of Health. He has been an avid supporter of GMOs and glyphosate and an unforgiving critic of biotech detractors. He has traveled across the country, and the world, giving speeches, making presentations, and working to convince regulators that independent academics such as himself view GMOs and glyphosate herbicides as perfectly safe. Through it all, he has proclaimed himself free from corporate control. But Chassy's veil of independence appeared quite thin when internal e-mails revealed multiple professional and financial links to Monsanto.

In one arrangement, Monsanto helped set Chassy up to run a website called Academics Review, which was designed to counter scientists, journalists, activists, and others who criticized GMOs and agrochemicals such as glyphosate. There was only one catch—Monsanto wanted to keep its involvement a secret. In a November 2010 e-mail laying out the plan, a period in which Chassy was still working at the university, Monsanto's chief of global scientific affairs, Eric Sachs, wrote to Chassy: "From my perspective the problem is one of expert engagement and that could be solved by paying experts to provide responses. . . . The key will be keeping Monsanto in the background so as not to harm the credibility of the information." In that same exchange, Sachs told Chassy that Monsanto had just "sent a gift of $10,000" to his university, "so the funds should be there."

Jay Byrne, president of the v-Fluence public relations firm and former head of corporate communications for Monsanto, told Chassy in a separate 2010 e-mail exchange that he was trying to move the Academics Review project forward and that he had a list of industry critics ready for Academics Review to target. He suggested "we work on the money (for all of us)." He told Chassy that the topic areas "mean money for a range of well heeled corporations."[16]

Chassy did not disappoint. Under his hand, the Academics Review site published several critical articles about individuals and organizations whose work did not support industry objectives, including the

IARC working group that classified glyphosate as a probable carcinogen. No disclosure was made of Monsanto's interests in, or support of, the website as it came out with the critical articles. But a look at tax filings makes the connections clear. Money was funneled through a nonprofit set up by the industry called the Council for Biotechnology Information (CBI), a group that states in government filings its goal is to "promote agricultural plant biotechnology through the exchange of information about its benefits." CBI directors included Phil Miller, global regulatory affairs vice president for Monsanto, as well as Dow's global affairs leader, Brad Shurdut, and DuPont's Jerry Flint, also a vice president for regulatory affairs. Academics Review received $300,000 from the CBI in 2014 and $350,000 in 2015, the records show. That was only a small portion of the millions of dollars the group spread around annually for "education, advocacy and other means" to groups in the United States, Mexico, and Canada.[17]

In addition to the website, Chassy helped Monsanto in many other ways. He coauthored a long article about Séralini, calling the study "fraudulent" and saying the work raised questions of "scientific misconduct."[18] Several e-mails from 2011 show that Chassy and Monsanto's Sachs, along with others in the industry, discussed ways to lobby the EPA against expanded regulation of biotech crops. And in a September 2011 e-mail exchange with people from Monsanto and industry, Chassy suggested how the biotech crop industry might "spin" a government report that found significant levels of glyphosate in air and water samples. Chassy referred to "anti-GM chemophobes" and told the group the "take home message" should be that the "mere presence of a chemical in an ecosystem or ecological niche is by itself meaningless. The antis always conveniently forget this."[19]

Chassy even traveled overseas to do Monsanto's bidding, in at least one case agreeing to a "mission" before he understood its objective, as seen in this excerpt from a January 2012 e-mail from Chassy to Sachs:

You originally asked if I would go to China and do what I did in Korea. You wanted to know if I was available and said you would explain later. One thing led to another and I am now going but we never did speak about the actual mission on China.

Where am I speaking? To whom? For how long? More importantly, what is the topic and is there an assigned title? What's really going on and what are the between the lines issues? Knowing the [answers] to all of these questions would really help me plan a talk.

Can we talk sometime before I start putting a talk together?[20]

In other exchanges, Chassy, Sachs, and Monsanto's John Swarthout, who led the company's scientific outreach and issues management, discussed what Chassy's China presentation should say, including changes made by Monsanto. Sachs instructed Swarthout to send slide decks to Chassy as material for him to use.

Monsanto's Hammond also asked Chassy for help creating short videos about the "safety of GM crops." In those e-mail exchanges, Chassy said he thought he could use university equipment to do the work and asked Hammond for a list of videos that "you think would be helpful."[21]

Chassy also was a regular contributor to an industry-funded promotional website called GMO Answers, where he wrote that research linking glyphosate to illnesses was flawed, again failing to disclose his ties to Monsanto. At the same time that some of this was going on, Monsanto money was flowing in Chassy's direction. It's unclear exactly how much money was involved, but several e-mails discussed financial payments. In one, Chassy told colleagues at the university that Monsanto had promised him the company was going to make a "substantial contribution" to his biotech account at the university.[22]

In a different e-mail exchange, Chassy asked Sachs about a contribution for the university foundation biotech fund. The Monsanto executive responded that he would "make a gift to the foundation right away" if it had not already been made.[23] Chassy said the check should be accompanied by a letter saying the check is "an unrestricted gift . . . in support of the biotechnology outreach and education activities of Professor Bruce M. Chassy."[24]

Chassy didn't disclose the financial relationships publicly. Instead, the payments were funneled through the University of Illinois Foundation, which does not have to report its funding, keeping the payments out of the public eye.[25]

Chassy said he did nothing unethical or improper in his work supporting Monsanto and the biotech crop industry. He said he was never asked to modify his independent views and was "never compensated in any way" for his expertise. Financial support from the private sector for public-sector research, education, and public outreach is not only appropriate, Chassy said, but needed. "As a public-sector research scientist, it was expected . . . that I collaborate with and solicit the engagement of those working in my field of expertise," Chassy stated on the Academics Review website in September 2015, the same month his relationship with Monsanto was revealed in an article in the *New York Times*.[26]

Monsanto also said there was nothing improper about the arrangement. But critics have argued the public is being misled by these types of covert connections. "These revelations regarding the connections are very important," said George Kimbrell, senior attorney with the Center for Food Safety, a nonprofit consumer advocacy group. "The basic disclosure that some academics and other 'neutral' commentators in the public sphere are actually paid operatives/working directly with the chemical industry rightly alarms the public, as they are being misled."[27]

Another U.S. professor who became a member of the inner circle of Monsanto academic allies was Kevin Folta of the University of Florida.

Folta, who holds a doctorate in molecular biology, was known as a strawberry expert, having helped lead a project to sequence the strawberry genome from 2007 to 2010. But Folta became a favored friend for Monsanto and its public relations teams around 2013 as they looked for people to help them combat GMO labeling efforts. Folta was eager and willing to assure the public that GMO crops were healthy and that glyphosate residues were not harmful.

Documents obtained by U.S. Right to Know revealed a series of arrangements between Monsanto and Folta to help Monsanto on its PR mission. In one e-mail, Folta told Monsanto he was "glad to sign on to whatever you like, or write whatever you like."[28] In fact, Folta was one of the nine professors Monsanto asked to write a policy brief in 2013. His assignment—to "provide examples of activist campaigns that spread false information that goes unchallenged." Folta was supposed to push a narrative that critics of GMO crops were undermining "worldwide efforts to ensure a safe, nutritious, plentiful and affordable food supply using responsible and sustainable agricultural practices."[29] Folta did as asked, the record shows.[30]

Folta was then, and is as of this writing, associate professor and chairman of the Horticultural Sciences Department at the university, so his credentials carry a lot of weight. A top executive with the Ketchum public relations firm made it clear how important Folta's work for the industry was, writing to him in May 2014: "Professors/researchers/scientists have a big white hat in this debate and support in their states, from politicians to producers. Keep it up!"[31]

Part of Folta's work with the industry included the use of his name and likeness on a pro-industry website called GMO Answers, funded by Monsanto, Dow, and other agrochemical and seed companies. Ketchum designed the site as a Q&A forum where academics such as Folta would appear to be relying on their expertise to address frequently asked questions about GMOs and agrochemicals. Ketchum said in one e-mail to

Folta that the website was "a new way to build trust, dialogue and support for biotech in agriculture."[32] But while the website stated that the answers came from Folta, they were actually written, at least in some cases, by the PR firm.[33]

Here is just one example of suggested text the PR firm wrote to post on the GMO Answers website attributed to Folta: "In the wild, the transfer of genes within and across species is fairly common, either through traditional reproduction (breeding) or through non-traditional means. Viruses and bacteria do this all the time, as do plants and animals. Human DNA, for instance, is full of viral genes."[34] The PR executive told Folta he was free to revise and use his own words. But in the public posting on the industry website, underneath a picture of a smiling Folta, not a word was changed.[35]

When IARC's classification of glyphosate's probable carcinogenicity hit the news, Folta was cited by GMO Answers as an "expert" on the issue, with a column under his name declaring glyphosate as "amazingly non-toxic to humans or any other animals." In all, Folta was cited as an expert on the corporate-run website more than seventy times from 2013 through 2015—all of this while he ostensibly was working for a taxpayer-funded public university.

The agrochemical and seed industry players were also paying for Folta to travel, make speeches, and give industry-friendly presentations. In August 2014, Monsanto agreed to provide an "unrestricted grant" of $25,000 for Folta to travel to several universities to "train" faculty, staff, and students about GMO agriculture. But again, keeping the ties a secret was part of the plan. Folta suggested that Monsanto send its money to a program within the nonprofit University of Florida Foundation that would allow the funding to be hidden from public scrutiny. The program was known as Special Help for Agricultural Research and Education, or SHARE. "If funded directly to the program as a SHARE contribution (essentially unrestricted funds) it is not . . . in a 'conflict-of-interest' account. In other words, SHARE contributions are not pub-licly noted," Folta told Monsanto. "This eliminates the potential con-cern of the funding organization influencing the message."[36]

After the *New York Times* revealed Folta's arrangements with Mon-santo, the university and Folta came under heavy public criticism and the university announced that the $25,000 was "re-allocated" to a Florida food pantry. Folta defended his work with Monsanto, saying the con-troversy was built on "manufactured" narratives. "I had an established, effective program that a company wanted to support," Folta said in a statement posted by the university. "Science can benefit from corpo-rate partnerships to foster efforts of scientific literacy, and that helps all of us."

Folta continues to be an active advocate for Monsanto and its prod-ucts, including glyphosate, and routinely makes written attacks on jour-nalists, scientists, and others who point to research that doesn't align with industry interests. He's criticized me on social media forums and in blog posts, writing that I am a "hideous human" and "disgusting." In one of a series of e-mails Folta wrote to me, he said that I was a "liar and manipulator." He also told me that he made disclosures about his ties to industry "to the level required" and says he "acknowledged it when it was relevant."

Even though he asserts he has done nothing wrong, Folta says that being caught in the public spotlight the way he was has taken a toll on his professional and emotional well-being. Folta said he has lost numer-ous opportunities because of the reports about his industry ties. "My hair started going grey and I aged a decade. . . . My breathing is slow and shallow, I don't sleep well. I'm forgetful. The toll has been harsh. My eyes swell with tears when I even think about what I have been through," he wrote on his website.[37]

The agricultural industry has cheered him on, awarding him the Borlaug CAST Communication Award in 2016—a designation to recognize those who "demonstrate a passionate interest in communicating the importance of agriculture to policymakers, the news media, and the public."[38]

Gary Ruskin, codirector of U.S. Right to Know, said that the pattern of corporate influence over American academics discovered by his nonprofit group is alarming because the hidden collaborations are aimed at papering over the health risks of products such as glyphosate. "Supposedly unbiased scientists have been degraded into corporate PR flaks," he said.[39]

Another favored strategy for the chemical industry has been to stake out spaces on social media, a vast Internet-based landscape where virtually anyone can blog or tweet or comment on any topic under the sun. Who would think that glyphosate would have its own Twitter account, for instance? But it does, with a long stream of positive messages about the agrochemical (with no disclosure as to who the account belongs to). Glyphosate is perhaps the world's first pesticide to have over 1,900 "followers" on a mainstream social media platform, where politicians, celebrities, and anyone else with a message to share can meet. Glyphosate's Twitter account was established in March 2015, the month IARC made its carcinogenic classification.

PR experts inside and outside Monsanto have also sought out bloggers to post articles that support GMOs and glyphosate on different consumer and health websites, including the popular WebMD, where readers turn for information on a range of health and nutrition topics.[40] "Mommy bloggers," women who write about parenting or related topics, are among the social media players Monsanto and its PR teams have recruited for positive commentary on agrochemical industry interests such as glyphosate and GMOs. Monsanto has ties to social media groups such as #Moms4GMOs and Science Moms, for instance. These groups post favorable industry information on an array of websites while appearing to be independent of industry influence.

Academics were also asked to write favorable blogs on WebMD without mentioning a Monsanto connection. Monsanto government affairs lead Lisa Drake laid it out for Folta in a January 2015 e-mail exchange. After wishing him a "Happy New Year," Drake asked Folta to submit a blog on the "safety and health of biotech to WebMD." She provided him with instructions on how to submit an article and asked him to be sure to "insert the word 'labeling' somewhere in the content in order to get search algorithms to pick it up." She underscored how hard Monsanto was working to get favorable content published: "Over the past six months, we have worked hard through third parties to insert fresh and current material on Web MD's website." Folta replied within a few minutes, "Can do! My pleasure."[41]

Anna Lappé, cofounder of the nonprofit Small Planet Institute, calls the tactics "stealth marketing techniques" that work "surreptitiously to shape public opinion." In an opinion piece she authored on the topic, Lappé said this:

> Sure, PR is an old game, but Big Ag is giving the age-old techniques of shaping public opinion a new, sneakier spin. Much of today's marketing happens behind the scenes and off the printed page—on the Web pages of blogs, on Twitter feeds and Facebook pages, through sponsored content and industry-funded webisodes and on the stages of big-ideas festivals.[42]

There are in fact small armies of industry promoters spread across social media, trolling for negative commentary and responding to any they find with fast retorts that back industry interests. Sometimes the connections between these social media players and certain corporations are clear-cut, sometimes not. But the social media circles have been growing in power and influence. Court documents state that one such strategy by Monsanto, called "Let nothing go," is designed to monitor social media postings and respond to any critical comments or articles about industry interests.[43]

The Center for Food Safety found out just how powerful the social media strategy could be when the organization scheduled a presentation in Honolulu, Hawaii, by author, activist, and Monsanto critic Vani Hari, who markets herself as Food Babe. Event organizers slated the presentation for September 2016 and offered free tickets to the public but asked that people who wanted to attend RSVP so they could be guaranteed a seat. In an effort to sabotage the event, a pro-Monsanto group that refers to itself as March Against Myths About Modification put out a social media call for help. The group asked Facebook followers to make large numbers of fake reservations so the event would appear sold out but would actually leave Hari speaking to a nearly empty hall. Leaders encouraged people to use fake names and create "disposable" e-mail addresses, even providing instructions on how to do so, to reserve the seats. More than 1,500 tickets were reserved this way under names like Harriett Tubman, Fraud Babe, and Susi Creamcheese. Facebook postings showed scores of people from around the world making fake reservations and joking about the deceit.[44] Organizers uncovered the scheme the day before the event and were able to cancel many of the fake reservations, opening up seats for valid reservations.

Hari said the events were jarring. "I choose to put my focus and energy on the willing—the people who want to hear about what's really in their food and how they can make healthy changes to their lifestyle. On the other hand, there are some serious detractors that do not want the truth about our food to be heard. They are working as agents for the biotech and chemical industry to prevent information about the risks of using chemicals like glyphosate that are coupled with GMOs to come to light."[45]

The March Against Myths group is just one of various organizations created, funded, or otherwise backed by agribusiness to tout its messages. In some cases, the links to industry are clear, while in other cases, they are harder to see. These front groups act essentially as echo chambers, citing each other as sources that reinforce industry positions with the veneer of expertise and impartiality. Their names often sound impressive and authoritative. Take, for instance, the American Council on Science and Health (ACSH), the group Monsanto positioned to help it promote the policy briefs by Folta, Juma, and the other academics. The ACSH was founded in 1978 and bills itself as a national non-profit education organization that supports "evidence-based science and medicine." It does not publicly disclose the range of corporate funding it relies on, but records obtained by journalists in 2013 reveal a money trail that leads to a number of chemical companies as well as prominent food and tobacco companies.[46] The group has been a vocal supporter of glyphosate, calling questions about its safety "ridiculous fearmongering."[47] The ACSH, not coincidentally, uses its website to promote the March Against Myths group, which tried to sabotage Hari's speech, and to attack people who raise questions about glyphosate's safety. The group wrote and featured a piece on its website accusing a *New York Times* reporter of "lying" when he authored an article about glyphosate concerns.[48]

Folta and other industry supporters similarly interfered with a speech planned for early 2016 in Houston by Thierry Vrain, a Canadian molecular biologist who has raised concerns about glyphosate and GMOs. Vrain was to deliver a lecture at the Houston Museum of Natural Science titled "The Poison in Our Food Supply." A few days beforehand, a storm of e-mails, phone calls, and social media messages, along with a blog piece written by Folta, assailed the museum for hosting the event, claiming Vrain lacked credibility. Many accused Vrain of practicing "junk science" and threatened to cancel their museum membership if it didn't ax the lecture. The museum president succumbed to the pressure and canceled the event. Organizers were able to find an alternative venue nearby and the evening lecture was held anyway, but the power of the industry cheerleaders was clear.[49]

In fact, there are many industry-backed organizations that often coordinate with the companies and their public relations arms to try to sway public opinion and push for favorable public policies. And, like the ACSH, they sound quite impressive. There is the International Life Sciences Institute, the U.S. Farmers and Ranchers Alliance, and the Alliance to Feed the Future. Records show the organizations all have received funding from Monsanto and numerous other food or chemical companies or corporate-funded trade groups. Monsanto created a group called America's Farmers out of whole cloth, and it formed and funded a group of dietitians specifically "to communicate with consumers who have questions about food and agriculture." Called Leaders Engaged in Advancing Dialogue (LEAD), the organization is made up of registered dietitians around the country who receive talking points from Monsanto and participate in events the company lines up. They are active both on the ground and across social media, protecting industry interests.

And in a very targeted move, a group called Campaign for Accuracy in Public Health Research was launched in early 2017 specifically to tear down the credibility of IARC for having classified glyphosate as possibly carcinogenic. The group, which called itself an "education and outreach initiative," declared its first mission was to "reform" IARC and "bring to light the deficiencies, misinformation and consequences" of IARC's findings.[50] And just who was behind this new group that aims to "promote credible, unbiased, and transparent science"? None other than the American Chemistry Council, whose membership includes the agrochemical industry heavyweights Monsanto, Dow, DuPont, and Bayer.

The industry hides behind such friendly sounding organizations, according to public health attorney Michele Simon, who wrote a detailed report in 2013 on industry front group activity. "The idea is to fool the media, policymakers, and general public into trusting these sources, despite their corporate-funded PR agenda," Simon said. "Industry spin is becoming more prevalent and aggressive."[51]

Glyphosate is such a critical moneymaker for the agrochemical industry that there are organizations devoted solely to the chemical. The Glyphosate Task Force, formed in Europe by a consortium of chemical companies including Monsanto, has significant influence as a provider of research data to regulators. It does not seek to appear independent of industry, nor does its counterpart in North America, the Joint Glyphosate Task Force. Still, the depths of their influence on regulators is often murky. When IARC made the glyphosate classification, both organizations decried IARC and sought to direct attention instead to a "Renewal Assessment Report," or RAR, produced by the German government in 2013 that concluded glyphosate was unlikely to pose a cancer risk to humans. That RAR recommended that the acceptable daily intake for glyphosate actually be increased by 67 percent because glyphosate was so safe. And because it was released by a government entity, the RAR appeared authoritative enough to counter IARC's findings. But few knew that RAR actually relied heavily on a dossier put together by the Glyphosate Task Force.[52] Though Monsanto's own work helped direct the findings, the company pointed to the RAR as independent and authoritative backing for glyphosate safety. And the public was none the wiser.

A group of six scientists and academic professors penned a letter in April 2017 calling for an end to the spin and the secrecy surrounding Monsanto's herbicide. "It is clear from the amount of time, effort, and money that the agrochemical industry has spent on trying to counter efforts to restrict the use of glyphosate, that they are quite concerned about lost profits from the sales of these products. Rather than cynically attempting to squeeze the last few dollars of profits from sales of chemicals that have been demonstrated to cause adverse health effects, the agrochemical industry should exert some corporate responsibility and open their concealed testing data regarding the safety of chemicals for public evaluation," the group wrote.[53]

CHAPTER 7

A Poisoned Paradise

The Hawaiian Islands have long been a draw for tourists from around the world. But the year-round climate of warm winds, sunshine, and ample moisture has also made the islands a hot spot for multinational agrochemical and seed companies, which see the tropical environment as an ideal testing ground for a range of new seeds and the chemicals used on them. Corn is the big seed crop, in high demand around the globe. And with the introduction of genetic engineering of corn and other seeds in the mid-1990s has come a broad expansion by the seed and chemical companies across Hawaiian farmland and broad use of glyphosate herbicides.

Monsanto Company, Dow Agrosciences, DuPont, Syngenta, and others snapped up leases for large swaths of property over the past several decades and transformed areas known for sugar and pineapple production into experimental field sites. By 2014, the chemical companies controlled more than 13,500 acres on the island of Kauai alone. Across the state, including on the islands of Maui, Molokai, and Oahu, the companies occupied about 25,000 of the state's 280,000 acres of agricultural land. With the year-round intensive crop work have come heavy applications of not just glyphosate but a range of pesticides, many with dangers that are better documented than those associated with glyphosate. The experiences of island residents illustrate how hard it can be to challenge chemically intensive agriculture and the powerful business interests behind it.

In addition to glyphosate, one pesticide of top concern is a bugkilling chemical called chlorpyrifos, which has been banned for residential use in the United States since the year 2000 because of its dangers. It is known to be highly toxic to fish and other aquatic life, and the U.S. Environmental Protection Agency (EPA) warns that it can overstimulate the human nervous system and can kill people at very high exposures. Even more worrisome, research by the Columbia Center for Children's Environmental Health found that children who had greater pre- and postnatal exposure to chlorpyrifos were more likely to have altered brain development and experience early childhood developmental delays, lower IQ scores, and a host of serious neurodevelopmental problems. The researchers said the findings suggest that neurotoxic effects of chlorpyrifos are "long term" and have important public health implications because of the fact that "widespread agricultural use . . . continues unabated."[1] And a review of the scientific literature published in February 2014 in the British journal *Lancet Neurology* cited chlorpyrifos among several commonly used chemicals that injure the developing brains of children.[2]

Still, chlorpyrifos has remained a key tool in agriculture, especially in production of corn, soybeans, fruit, and many types of vegetables, such as broccoli, cauliflower, and brussels sprouts. It's been used regularly by the chemical companies on the Hawaiian Islands, and the companies have fought mightily to keep using it despite the research on its dangers to children and others. The EPA proposed in October 2015 revoking all tolerances for chlorpyrifos, essentially banning it for any agricultural use, but only after being sued by environmentalists who argued the chemical is highly dangerous to both people and wildlife.[3] Despite the evidence of harm, Dow and others in the chemical industry protested the EPA moves, and the chemical remains on the market as a restricted use pesticide, or RUP, as of this writing.

Other chemicals used on island test fields include the herbicides atrazine and paraquat, both big sellers for agrochemical giant Syngenta. Studies have linked atrazine to endocrine disruption, miscarriage, birth defects, and cancer, and it has been banned in the European Union since 2003. And even though Switzerland-based Syngenta has been the largest producer of paraquat, the chemical is banned in that country because of links to Parkinson's disease, other neurological disorders, and cancer. Both are still allowed in the United States, though regulators have acknowledged the potential risks. Another pesticide used on the islands is methomyl, introduced by DuPont in 1968, which has similarly been shown to be problematic for humans and animals. The EPA has restricted its use because of the dangers. In fact, at least seven heavily used pesticides on the islands are so dangerous that their use is supposed to be tightly restricted per EPA requirements. More than 906,000 pounds of these RUPs was sold statewide in 2014, according to state data.[4] The state does not collect similar data on general use pesticides, such as glyphosate.

For residents of the Hawaiian Islands, the combination of chemicals has formed what many fear is a toxic soup poisoning their piece of paradise. And sadly, there is some evidence their fears could be well-founded. Alongside the climbing chemical use have come a range of reported health problems, including suspected poisoning episodes from spraying of pesticides near schools and homes and unusual rates of birth defects, cancers, and illnesses reported by medical practitioners. One group of doctors told lawmakers in 2013 that they were seeing more miscarriages than usual, abnormally high rates of very severe gout in otherwise healthy people, high rates of patients with respiratory problems, hormonal changes in patients causing excessive facial and body hair on women, recurring nosebleeds in children, and patients reporting a persistent metallic taste in their mouth. That physicians' group, from the island of Kauai, cited statistics that they said showed birth defects occurring at ten times the national rate. In a July 2013 letter to lawmakers, the doctors wrote:

> We have no direct evidence of a specific correlation between these unique variances in the health of some of our patients with the current or past agricultural practices but we do have a high level of suspicion that a strong correlation exists between the two.
>
> . . . We all share a deep concern for the health of our patients and the concern of what may be happening to our community by being exposed to this unique cocktail of experimental and restricted use pesticides on an almost daily basis.[5]

The fears are most pronounced on Kauai, the oldest of the Hawaiian Islands and affectionately known by its population of roughly 68,000 as the "Garden Isle" for its fertile soil and lush beauty. Kauai boasts emerald valleys, tropical rain forests, cascading waterfalls, and jagged cliffs thousands of feet high. But in recent years, the west side of the island has become known primarily for the intensive agrochemical industry presence there. BASF, Syngenta, DuPont, and Dow have made the land their own, testing an array of new crops and dousing them with a variety of chemicals, including RUPs such as chlorpyrifos and the less restricted glyphosate.

Some residents now call the west side of Kauai the "poison valley" and say they must constantly clean their houses of reddish dust and keep windows closed to avoid toxic vapors and chemical odors that waft through neighborhoods on brisk island breezes. Several residents of the town of Waimea sued DuPont over the chemical use and the impact on their homes. A jury awarded the residents $500,000 in 2015, finding that DuPont failed to follow good management practices on its fields.

On the other side of Waimea, the fears have focused on work by Syngenta that involves the spraying of pesticides in an area that abuts a middle school, a health clinic, and a veteran's hospital. Students at the school were evacuated twice, in 2006 and 2008, and taken to hospitals with flu-like symptoms that many townspeople blamed on the agro-chemical companies and their pesticide use. Syngenta contended the odors were caused by stinkweed, not pesticides. A government probe was unable to provide definitive answers as to what harmed the school-children but did find traces of chlorpyrifos and the insecticide bifen-thrin in air samples at the middle school.[6] Bifenthrin is another RUP and is deemed by the EPA to be a possible human carcinogen.

Another alarm bell rang when ten Syngenta employees were rushed to a local hospital on Kauai in January 2016 after walking onto a field too soon after it had been sprayed with chlorpyrifos. Company man-agement blamed the workers, saying they had strayed into a field where they were not scheduled to work. But the EPA sued Syngenta's Hawaii operation for failing to notify the workers of the danger and ordered the company to pay a fine of $4.9 million.

As signs of harm have mounted, worried Kauai residents have pushed to learn exactly how much of the agrochemicals are being used and where. One analysis of government pesticide databases and data from the Hawaii Department of Agriculture released in 2014 showed that the agrochemical industry was applying pesticides at higher rates on Kauai than the application rates on most U.S. farms. That report described the west side of Kauai as "one of the most toxic chemical environments in all of American agriculture."[7] Worried residents have asked for buffer zones between the pesticide spraying and schools and homes, but the pesticide companies disputed the findings of excessive pesticide use and have opposed any efforts that might limit their work.

For longtime Kauai doctor Lee Evslin, addressing the pesticide concerns on the island, where he and his wife have lived for more than thirty-five years and raised four children, has become, in his words, "an important battle."

Evslin was never one to seek out political involvement. He was content to spend his life as a physician with a specialty in caring for children. He first used his medical expertise to establish a neonatal intensive care unit on Guam before moving in 1979 to Kauai, where he built a career that included a private pediatric practice and a fifteen-year stint as administrator of a local hospital. But the rising concerns, and the tactics chosen by the pesticide companies to protect their work on the islands, have left him "appalled" and active in efforts to rein in the pesticide use.[8]

Evslin's outrage came after he spent fifteen months working with several other doctors and scientists on a joint fact-finding group formed by the state and local governments to gather data on the pesticide concerns. The group was called upon by government leaders to determine "if agricultural pesticide usage on Kaua'i is as dangerous and damaging as critics asserted or as safe and innocuous as the biotechnology companies claimed."[9] (Two representatives from the agrochemical industry— one from Dow and one from DuPont—resigned from the fact-finding group after the draft report was issued. The two complained the report was biased and not based on facts.)

That group's final report, issued in May 2016, found that the big seed companies applied an estimated 36,240 pounds, or 18.1 tons, of RUPs over a twenty-month period from December 2013 to July 2015. The group also found that the rate of RUP use on the island was generally higher than that on mainland farms, up to three times higher. The group said there was not enough information to conclude whether pesticide use by the seed companies played a role in health problems of Kauai residents, however. The group said more research and data were needed to draw firm conclusions about a causal relationship.[10] A separate report by the state found the incidence of cancer on Kauai was generally the same or even lower than for the state overall, and there are conflicting findings on the reports of other diseases as well.

But even without definitive causation evidence of human health problems tied to the pesticide use, Evslin came away more convinced than ever that the pervasiveness of the agrochemicals lays a dangerous path for the future of the island. "It is wrong what they are doing," he said of the pesticide industry's reluctance to make changes that might address concerns.

Evslin has specific worries about glyphosate, given the growing evidence of its ties to cancer and its common and widespread use, which leaves residues in food, water, air, and our bodies. "We all have a level of glyphosate in our bodies at all times," he said. "I can't imagine we were designed to have constant low levels of glyphosate in our bodies. Clearly, glyphosate in our food is not a good thing. The more I get involved in this, the more angry I become."

Many Kauai residents also are angry, and the island has become a political and legal battleground between those who want to rein in the pesticide companies and the industry and its allies who are determined to defend their work, which translates to economic gains for the state through lease income, taxes, and jobs.

The citizen uprising, as some describe it, reached a fever pitch in 2013 with efforts to force restrictions on the seed and chemical companies. A ten-page ordinance introduced in June of that year by Kauai County Council member Gary Hooser was seen as a first, though imperfect, step to try to get a handle on the pesticide use. The measure, House Bill 2491, required companies to disclose their pesticide use and the types of genetically engineered crops they were growing; set a 500-foot pesticide-free buffer zone around schools, hospitals, neighborhoods, and bodies of water; and called for a temporary moratorium on the experimental use and commercial production of genetically modified organisms (GMOs) until the county could conduct a health and environmental assessment. It also prohibited open-air testing of experimental pesticides and GMO crops.

By August 2013, the bill had become sharply divisive, drawing large crowds to public meetings and pitting people who worried about pesticide-related health and environmental problems against others who worried the restrictions might drive the agrochemical companies off the island, hurting the economy and triggering job losses. An estimated 4,000 island residents staged a march in support of the bill that September before a county council vote, but the bill was watered down in committee meetings, stripped of all but the buffer zones, the assessment, and the disclosure requirements for GMO and pesticide use. Prohibitions on open-air testing of experimental pesticides and crops fell away, and the temporary moratorium was also dropped from the bill.

The full council approved the revised bill, then known as Ordinance 960, only to have it vetoed by Kauai's mayor, Bernard Carvalho, who agreed with a pesticide industry argument that it was the state's role to regulate pesticides and GMOs, not the island's, which operates under a county government. The county council disagreed and overrode the mayor's veto in November 2013, but its victory was short-lived because less than two months later Syngenta, DuPont, and a company affiliated with Dow called Agrigenetics sued to block the new law from taking effect. A federal judge agreed with the agrochemical companies in August 2014, saying the county didn't have the authority to regulate the companies' actions. But the residents of Kauai would not stop pressing for action. In October of that year, a group of them reached out for help to the federal Centers for Disease Control and Prevention (CDC), asking for a public health assessment that would seek to determine if people near the island test fields were in fact being exposed to harmful pesticide levels as suspected and what impact the pesticide use was having on human health. The petition stated the group's position this way:

Great health concerns exist in the community because of the intense agricultural practices utilizing a large amount and variety of pesticides being used in experimental conditions near some communities. Recent environmental studies have identified the existence of these agro-chemicals both in the air and the open waterways near where people live, work and go to school. In addition, anecdotal evidence indicates that the community may be experiencing some adverse and an abnormally high number of health issues that may be attributable to the chemicals being used.[11]

Ileana Arias, head of the CDC's Agency for Toxic Substances and Disease Registry (ATSDR), denied the request, saying such an investigation would be "challenging." She said the ATSDR had reviewed available data on a range of relevant topics and found the data either lacking or indicative of no association between health problems and pesticide residues. She acknowledged there was no information available about the amount of general use pesticides applied, such as glyphosate, and acknowledged that companies appear to be applying one to three times the amounts of RUPs per acre on Kauai than on corn acreage on the U.S. mainland. But even though the data points "suggest Kaua'i residents might be exposed to more pesticides than U.S. mainland populations," Arias said if other factors are taken into account, such as weather and varying times and locations of applications, "the opportunity for residents of Kaua'i west side communities to be exposed to pesticides [is] probably no different from the U.S. mainland."

She also said existing cancer data did not warrant concern, nor did existing research on birth defects. Only a few published articles supported an association between pesticide exposure and an increased rate of birth defects, including those of concern on Kauai, and many of those studies were "not very robust" and had "significant limitations." Arias summed up her decision this way:

ATSDR is not able to demonstrate scientifically whether people near agricultural fields in Kaua'i west side communities are being exposed to pesticides at levels of health concern. Accordingly, ATSDR will not conduct any [additional] public health assessment activities specifically about the pesticide use on the crop fields at Kaua'i, Hawaii.

The agency did say it would work with the Hawaii Department of Health to "provide the local professional healthcare community with an opportunity to learn more about environmental contaminants and their potential health impacts."[12]

Even as the Kauai effort was floundering, a burgeoning citizens' movement was mounting on the island of Maui to try to reign in Monsanto and Dow, which both had research farms on the island. Monsanto at the time was employing about 365 people on 3,000 acres it owned or leased within Maui County, while a Dow unit had about 100 workers on about 420 acres. Concerned Maui County residents had taken photos and submitted evidence to state regulators that they said showed glyphosate being sprayed frequently in areas near schoolchildren and along commonly traveled public roads and pathways.

Shortly after the law in Kauai was overturned, voters in Maui approved a moratorium on the cultivation of genetically engineered crops until scientific studies were conducted on their safety and benefits. But one week after the measure passed, in November 2014, Monsanto and Dow filed suit to block the law and invalidate the voter-approved measure. Again, the companies found victory through the courts. "If effective, the referendum will have significant negative consequences for the local economy, Hawaii agriculture and our business on the island," Monsanto said in a statement issued when the lawsuit was filed.[13]

Residents of the Big Island of Hawaii had a similar experience, pursuing an ordinance in 2013 that would restrict the seed companies' ability to operate, only to see the effort fail in the face of corporate opposition. Mark Phillipson, an executive of the Swiss seed and agrochemical company Syngenta, explained why being able to work on the Hawaiian Islands is so important to the industry: "Almost any corn seed sold in the U.S. touches Hawaii somewhere," he told the *New York Times.*[14]

The companies have seen strong support from many who say the seed business is vital to the economy, contributing more than $200 million and thousands of jobs. The Hawaii Crop Improvement Association, which acts as a trade association for the seed and chemical companies, disputes that there is any credible statistical health information to support claims of birth defects and other health problems tied to the pesticide use.

Nevertheless, people are still scared—both about pesticide use generally and about glyphosate in particular. On the main island, the Hawaii State Senate held a hearing in March 2014 to examine glyphosate use and possible dangers. The prevalence of the pesticide was underscored by a study conducted by the state's health and agriculture departments, with help from the U.S. Geological Survey. The study sampled seven streambed sites around the state and found glyphosate residues in every one. Atrazine was also commonly found statewide. In all, researchers found that surface water samples collected from twenty-four sites around the islands showed at least one pesticide in every location.[15]

A year later, in 2015, the Hawaii County Council took up a bill to ban the spraying of glyphosate and other pesticides on government grounds. The bill's sponsor, Kohala council member Margaret Wille, said that concerns about Roundup needed to be addressed. The bill's goal was to "decrease the exposure of humans, birds, animals, beneficial insects and aquatic life to toxic herbicides in public places, roadways and waterways." Such a measure was needed because of "more and more evidence that cumulative exposure to toxic herbicides, including those containing glyphosate, is harmful to people as well as to land and water ecosystems."[16]

As might be expected, Wille's proposed ordinance was fiercely resisted by public officials and industry supporters, who argued that giving up Roundup would be too expensive and was unnecessary. Wille pulled the bill when she realized it appeared doomed, but she continued pushing for support and reintroduced it in 2016. Still, the bill failed to advance amid stiff opposition from industry representatives and public officials.

Fighting the various measures turned into a multimillion-dollar effort for Monsanto and other agrochemical industry players as they poured money into litigation and into lobbying lawmakers and the public. The industry spent approximately $8 million on just one campaign—trying to stop the Maui County GMO moratorium ballot initiative, marking the highest amount ever expended on a Hawaii election issue.[17] Throughout the state, the industry flexed its muscle with radio and television ads, television infomercials, mailers, and Internet campaigns to oppose restrictions on its island activities. Industry-friendly scientists such as Kevin Folta also traveled to Hawaii to make presentations about the safety of the agrochemical industry activities.

Kauai County Council member Hooser, who became somewhat of a legendary figure for fighting the agrochemical industry on his home island, began the quest simply as a response to concerns raised by constituents and never expected the issue to spiral into the drawn-out and highly charged battle it became. He was surprised when he first approached industry representatives to ask for data on pesticide usage only to be rebuffed. And over time, he said, he witnessed tactics that he thought were unethical, such as chemical companies paying people to hold places in line outside council meetings so that industry representatives could fill public hearing rooms, or filling buses with employees to show up at council meetings to oppose the measure. He also said he was personally threatened and vilified by supporters of agrochemical interests. Some of the threats became so alarming that he reported them to local authorities, he said.

"At first I just thought maybe we needed closer regulation, but after seeing these companies up close and personal—I want them gone. They are bad news," Hooser told me. "They act like, and say, they are highly regulated. But they aren't. I've asked them repeatedly to tell me how much glyphosate they're using. And they refuse to do it. And they always say no one is going to be sick, but that is not true. I've come to realize there is very little accountability, and I'm concerned about my community."[18]

Hooser has lived on the islands since moving to Honolulu with his family in the 1970s as a high school student. He worked odd jobs, moved to South Africa briefly to pursue the woman who would become his wife, and then returned to the islands, where he settled on Kauai and ran first a video arcade and then a series of small businesses, including a local magazine. He described his decision to run for public office after he turned forty as a "midlife crisis," prompted in part by a desire to help support certain social issues, such as same-sex marriage. He served on the county council and then spent eight years in the Hawaii State Senate before returning to the council, where he started hearing from constituents about pesticide companies.

"This was a wide cross section of the community, not just environmentalists who were concerned about what was going on along the west side of Kauai," he said. "The straw that broke the camel's back for me was when I found out there were about 150 residents suing DuPont Pioneer. This is unheard of, to sue the largest employer. The combined concern made me aware that I needed to do something, at least start asking questions." Hooser said he arranged meetings with Dow, BASF, DuPont, and Syngenta but was unable to get straight answers about what types and amounts of pesticides were being used.

"They don't want anyone to tell them what to do. But the more they've fought and pushed and lied, the more committed I've become to fight them," said Hooser. "There is no doubt in my mind that we are on the right side of history in this issue."

In the spring of 2015, Hooser traveled to Basel, Switzerland, to address shareholders at Syngenta's annual meeting, held at the company's headquarters. He was allowed to address the shareholders and present them with a petition, asking them to compel Syngenta to "honor the laws of our community." Another representative from Kauai who traveled with Hooser was able to video record the first few minutes of his speech before a security guard ordered her to stop. "We are very, very concerned about our community and the impacts that Syngenta has in our small community," Hooser told the shareholders. But his plea was unsuccessful.

Hooser and his wife raised two children on the island and became grandparents in the fall of 2016, giving Hooser added motivation to work for pesticide reductions. Hooser lost his seat on the county council in the November 2016 elections, but he has continued to work for what he calls a "common quest" to improve and protect the environment.

"This has been a life-changing experience for many people," he said. "With the birth of my grandson, it really has made me think long and hard about this more than ever before. The issue to me actually is about corporate greed and what it is doing to the world."[19]

Another longtime Hawaii resident who is worried about the pesticides is lawyer Paul Achitoff. After graduating from Harvard University and then Columbia Law School, Achitoff spent eleven years practicing business and environmental litigation in Los Angeles and Honolulu, defending companies and individuals, including those who were breaking environmental laws and harming consumers. The work didn't sit well with his conscience, and Achitoff eventually switched sides, joining the nationwide nonprofit public interest law group Earthjustice in 1994. There, he built a career protecting endangered species, migratory birds, and the health of waterways. As managing attorney for Earth-justice's mid-Pacific office in Honolulu, Achitoff became one of the key legal experts participating in the islands' efforts to understand and address pesticide risks.

Like others engaged in the fight, Achitoff sees a lack of government-collected data, and a lack of interest in collecting that data, as a real barrier to understanding.

"Neither the department of health, nor the department of agriculture, nor any other government agency has bothered to collect such data. And since none has committed to doing so in the future, we can expect that residents and workers will continue to at best worry and at worst get sick while industry and government continue to pretend that there's nothing to worry about," he said.[20]

Some state lawmakers did try to push through a measure that would have required monthly disclosure of the types and amounts of pesticides being used and where they were being used across the state, somewhat similar to the action Kauai tried and failed to implement. California has had such requirements for more than two decades, and the data are plugged into a map so residents can see what types of pesticides are being sprayed near them. The data also help researchers to study whether there are correlations between types and amounts of chemicals being sprayed and reported health problems. Researchers at the University of California, Berkeley, were able to use the state-gathered data in a 2011 study that found exposure to a combination of paraquat and the fungicide maneb increased the risk of Parkinson's disease.[21]

A bill to set up a similar data collection program in Hawaii passed through the state senate but stalled in the house after agricultural industry representatives argued that the reporting requirements would be overly burdensome on their businesses.

Achitoff sees the lack of data collection as only one part of a much bigger problem. All the local efforts to rein in pesticide use have lost in court on the basis of assertions that it is up to state and federal governments, not localities, to oversee pesticide use. But the state has failed for years to provide such oversight, according to Achitoff. Government records obtained by Achitoff through the Freedom of Information Act show that the state has fallen far behind in its inspection and enforcement duties, failing to follow up on years of required examinations of possible pesticide use violations. The EPA noted as much in reviews of the Hawaii Department of Agriculture (HDOA) in 2013 and 2015, citing approximately 700 inspection files in need of review, some dating back to 2008.

Achitoff filed a formal complaint with the EPA in August 2016 over the HDOA's lack of oversight, saying the state's "lackadaisical approach to enforcement allows pesticide users to imagine that careless practices, or even knowing violations, have no consequences." The state's "refusal to take seriously the effects of pesticides on health and the environment, also have created a crisis of confidence, with Hawaii residents understandably convinced the foxes are guarding the henhouse," Achitoff told the EPA in his August 2016 complaint.[22]

In response, the EPA acknowledged the problems and said it would work to secure additional funding to provide near-term help for the HDOA and it planned to keep a close eye on the state's progress in reducing its backlog and improving oversight.

Achitoff also registered a formal complaint with the EPA and the U.S. Department of Justice alleging that the lack of regulation by Hawaii authorities violated the civil rights of native Hawaiians by causing adverse impacts on the people. He cited many examples to back his claim, including data showing that restrictions on pesticide discharges into a drainage ditch system on West Kauai were lifted in 2015, a move that translated into violations of the Clean Water Act:

Millions of gallons of drainage waters containing toxic pollutants flow through the system and populated areas, and into the nearshore ocean waters, without any regulation or monitoring. . . . Testing has shown the presence of harmful pesticides including atrazine, chlorpyrifos, glyphosate, and metolachlor in the drainage ditches, in addition to many other pollutants.

These unregulated and unmonitored discharges are of particular concern since Native Hawaiians gather limu and fish in these areas. The open ditches are not fenced off or marked with warning signs to prevent children from playing in them. The outfalls funnel polluted waters into areas popular for fishing surfing, swimming, and boating.[23]

It's all intensely frustrating for Achitoff, who believes corporate profits are taking precedence over people's lives. "The genetic engineering companies have a very big role here, and they don't care about things like sustainability, the environment, or growing food for the people on the islands," he said. "They think of farming in terms of inputs and outputs and the bottom line."[24]

~

The corporations and the people of Hawaii are in for a long battle, according to Peter Adler, a consultant who specializes in mediation and conflict resolution. Adler helped lead the joint fact-finding group on Kauai and has stayed engaged in the debate. Advocates continue to push for more disclosure, more research, and more caution related to pesticide use.

"This battle is not going to go away," he said. "This is a political storm. The winds are shifting around a bit, but it's not clear where the winds are going to blow next."[25]

CHAPTER 8
Angst in Argentina

American farmland has long been the largest market for genetically engineered seeds and the glyphosate herbicides used on them, but the United States is by no means the only country to have adopted the new technology with open arms. Farmers in Argentina started using genetically engineered seeds about the same time farmers in the United States did, after regulators in Argentina approved Monsanto Company's Roundup Ready soybeans in 1996. Soy production soared over the next decade as farmers who previously had been tending to grass-fed cattle, growing rice and potatoes, or running dairy farms shifted their focus to growing soybeans. Many farmers plowed up pastures to become part of what was billed as a biotech revolution. Because the beans tolerated direct sprays of glyphosate herbicide, controlling weeds was easier than ever, and, like the Americans, Argentine farmers quickly became eager buyers of both the specialty seeds and the glyphosate chemicals. The timing was perfect. Rising demand for protein—translation: meat—was fueling strong global demand for soy needed to feed livestock that would end up on dinner plates around the world. Argentina soon became the world's third-largest soybean supplier, and genetically modified soybeans became Argentina's most important export. Argentine farmers adopted biotech cotton and corn as well, with roughly 24 million acres of the nation's farmland planted with biotech seeds by 2014, most of which were designed to be sprayed with glyphosate.

As in the United States, aggressive use of glyphosate year after year on farm fields led to a rise in glyphosate-resistant weeds, spurring many farmers to use more and more of the herbicide, often alongside other chemicals, to fight back. According to data from the Food and Agriculture Organization of the United Nations, total pesticide use in Argentina rose by 90 percent between 1997, when the country was beginning to adopt the new type of farming, and 2011, when it was well established. Use of herbicides, including glyphosate, rose by 185 percent during that time frame. And, just as in the United States, concerns for human health and for the environment have emerged.

By 2002, less than a decade after Roundup Ready soybeans were launched, some doctors in soybean-growing areas started reporting a suspicious rise in health problems in their patients, including birth defects and several types of cancer. People living in rural soybean-growing areas were notably affected, with sharply increased rates of miscarriage as well, according to scientists and physicians. In Santa Fe, cancer rates were documented at two to four times higher than the national average. In Chaco, regional birth reports showed a quadrupling of congenital defects, from 19.1 per 10,000 to 85.3 per 10,000 in the decade after GMO crops and glyphosate took hold in Argentina. Doctors there found that more of the diseases and birth defects occurred in villages near the soy fields than near cattle ranches.[1] A government study also noted troubling levels of agrochemical residues in the soil and drinking water in certain areas, with roughly 12 million people living in the country's farm belt potentially at risk.

Worried parents started complaining to government officials about their children getting sick; they blamed the increased illness on intensive chemical use on GMO soybean fields and cornfields surrounding their towns and villages. As did the people of Hawaii, many Argentines sought tighter controls on how and where glyphosate and other agrochemicals were used—demanding that schools and neighborhoods be protected. Protesters, including doctors, parents, and scientists, argued that liberal spraying of pesticides near populated areas, particularly aerial spraying by planes, was clearly dangerous to people, both through the nearly invisible chemical drifts that traveled on breezes off the fields and through residues that lingered in water and soil.

By 2006, the voices of protest were loud enough to convince a division of Argentina's agriculture ministry to recommend adding warning labels to glyphosate mixtures; the labels would have advised users to spray the chemicals only in farm areas, far away from homes and other well-populated areas. Agrochemical companies pushed back, and the ministry failed to fully implement the recommendation. Concerns persisted, and by 2009 President Cristina Fernández de Kirchner was motivated to set up a commission to study agrochemical impacts on human health. The commission found there was a need for more controls over herbicide mixing and use and for more studies of formulations containing glyphosate. But both U.S. authorities and the agrochemical industry argued that glyphosate and the other chemicals used on the soy fields and cornfields were important for maximizing production and had been shown to be safe to use on the fields. Argentine authorities found themselves caught between the farming and chemical industry interests, who had profits to protect, and protesters, who claimed their very lives were at stake.

For one small and mostly poor community in Argentina's central farming belt, a town called Ituzaingó, the concerns turned poignantly painful as children there began to fall ill with what seemed to be increasing frequency after the area adopted intensive production of GMO soy. One Ituzaingó woman, Sofia Gatica, felt driven to act after her newborn daughter died of kidney failure in 1999. Gatica, a working-class mother of three, had only a high school education, but she was convinced her daughter's death was tied to her own exposure while pregnant to the active spraying of agrochemicals on the soy fields that surrounded her community. Gatica began to knock on door after door around her town, talking with other mothers about their children and curious ailments. She learned that she was not alone in fearing the chemicals from the farm fields. Gatica and several other women eventually formed a group called the Mothers of Ituzaingó and filed multiple complaints with local leaders, protesting corporate influence in what the group called the poisoning of their town's population of 5,000 residents.

The complaints from Gatica's group and others got the attention of regulators and helped spur studies that revealed residues of glyphosate and the insecticide endosulfan in and around people's homes in the Ituzaingó area. Both chemicals were commonly sprayed from the air onto area farm fields, a practice that many feared encouraged the pesticide's drift into the town. At that time, glyphosate was touted as safe, but endosulfan was considered especially toxic and dangerous to human health and the environment.

By 2008, government officials were so concerned that the nation's minister of health began an investigation of the impact of the pesticide use in Ituzaingó. Research revealed that traces of herbicide and insecticide were detected in the blood of 80 percent of the children from the Ituzaingó area. Data also showed that cancer cases had jumped by 50 percent, to 300 from 2001 to 2009, an incidence rate forty-one times the national average. The evidence of harm was enough to lead authorities to pass a local prohibition on aerial spraying in Ituzaingó at a distance of 2,500 meters (a little more than a mile and a half) or less from residences.

Gatica was honored as an environmental hero for her work and was named a 2012 recipient of the international Goldman Environmental Prize. In a videotaped interview conducted as part of the award program,

Gatica explained why she was so motivated: "For me, these soybeans mean only destruction and death. When they spray the soy, they also spray us. At first I didn't associate my daughter's illness with pesticide spray. I felt horrible. It was very hard on me." Eventually, she said, she realized her family was not alone. "What happened in Ituzaingó is a hidden genocide because they poison you slowly and silently."

Gatica said she was warned against going after the pesticide industry, told to "stop messing with the soy," and even threatened once at gun-point, ordered to stop her anti-pesticide protests.[2] Gatica said many of her neighbors also were angry with her for her work, complaining their home values were diminished by the attention she drew to the area's health problems.

Use of the insecticide endosulfan is now banned in Argentina, and in many countries around the world, after representatives from 127 gov-ernments added it to a United Nations list of pollutants to be eliminated because of its ability to cause reproductive and developmental damage in both animals and humans. Use of glyphosate has continued, how-ever. Gatica has called for it to be banned as well and has continued her protest work.[3]

The efforts in Ituzaingó garnered international attention, but it is just one community among many around the country that are pushing back against agrochemicals. Some doctors are so concerned that they have formed a group called Doctors of Fumigated Towns to investigate and raise awareness of what they believe are clear connections between agricultural pesticide applications and a decline in health of people liv-ing near farming areas.

When the group held its first meeting at the National University of Córdoba in August 2010, 160 doctors from ten provinces and dozens of towns showed up to share stories of alarming health trends among their patients. It was at that meeting that the doctors began to grasp the potential magnitude of the problem as one after another they laid out evidence of curious birth defects, cancers, reproductive problems, and respiratory ailments.[4]

The group was founded and coordinated by Dr. Medardo Ávila Vázquez, a pediatrician and neonatologist from the medical faculty of the National University of Córdoba. Ávila Vázquez explained why he was driven to get involved: "The change in how agriculture is produced has brought, frankly, a change in the profile of diseases. We've gone from a pretty healthy population to one with a high rate of cancer, birth defects, and illnesses seldom seen before."[5]

In its 2011 meeting, also held at the university in Córdoba, the group called on lawmakers to restrict pesticide use and prohibit aerial spraying. The group blamed the "multinational laboratories" for promoting a growing use of dangerous pesticides. In that meeting, the organization issued a formal declaration of what it said were "certainties":

> That the effect on health in populations located in areas subjected to constant fumigation in Argentina is considerable, and that the situation is worsening day by day, with more frequent cases of severe diseases such as cancer, spontaneous abortions, fertility disorders and births of children with congenital malformations.
>
> That different health conditions, such as respiratory, endocrine, neurological, hematological and psychological conditions, are much more frequent in populations systematically sprayed as a result of the current agro-industrial model of production.
>
> That the use of pesticides is increasing every year. . . .
>
> That as much as we would have wanted a different reality, the only truth is what we know today: the current agricultural production system is responsible for causing these health problems, as well as other serious ecological and sociological problems not mentioned here.[6]

By November 2015, the group had honed in on glyphosate as a key culprit in health problems after the International Agency for Research on Cancer's classification of the chemical's probable carcinogenicity. Glyphosate and other agrochemicals were contributing to increases in "spontaneous abortions and congenital malformations, endocrine problems such as hypothyroidism, neurological disorders or cognitive development problems" and rising cancer rates, the group said. "There is no doubt that the massive and growing exposure to pesticides modified the disease profile of Argentine rural populations and that cancer is the leading cause of death among them," the organization said.[7]

About 500 miles from Córdoba, in Aviá Teraí, a volunteer network of doctors, lawyers, and scientists also has been working to convince authorities to put tighter controls on pesticide spraying, particularly from the air. The town is rustic and lacks running water, which leaves residents to rely on rainwater or other sources that can be contaminated with pesticides. The paucity of clean water also makes it more challenging to wash food and clothing, which can be contaminated by the chemicals used on the nearby fields. Many children suffer from an array of ailments, including odd hairy moles and nonmalignant tumors on their faces and bodies.[8]

The connections between agrochemicals and health problems in Argentina grabbed the global spotlight again in 2013 when the Associated Press (AP) published an investigation documenting the parallel phenomena of rising disease and rising use of agrochemicals in that country's farm belt. Overall, Argentine farmers were applying more than twice as much agrochemical concentrate per acre as U.S. farmers were, an AP analysis of government and pesticide industry data found. And the news outlet documented dozens of cases around the country where agrochemicals were being used or stored improperly, increasing the exposure risks. Those applying the chemicals were mixing glyphosate with chemicals such as 2,4-D, an herbicide associated with the defoliant called Agent Orange, used on jungles during the Vietnam War, according to the news investigation. Children were noted with a range of birth defects that included malformed brains, exposed spinal cords, blindness and deafness, other neurological damage, and strange skin problems.[9]

Government officials largely dismissed the issue, citing "misinformation," and said citizens were simply "dizzy and confused." Monsanto had a similar reaction, downplaying the health concerns and saying it could not be held responsible if people applying glyphosate or other chemicals failed to use proper safety precautions. Glyphosate is far less toxic than other types of pesticides that it has replaced, the company said. And, Monsanto said, Argentines should recognize that they have benefited greatly from the farming system Monsanto's products helped create because grain output has more than tripled since 1990.

But critics of the pesticide use say the documented health problems should not be ignored and that applications of glyphosate—used at the high volumes seen in the past two decades—must be considered more carefully. They cite the research of Andrés Carrasco, who found severe malformations from glyphosate in chicken and frog embryos significant enough to warrant further study.

Carrasco's work, which was first reported in the local press in the spring of 2009 and then published in a scientific journal in August 2010, became a rallying cry for critics of Monsanto and its glyphosate-based Roundup Ready cropping system. Carrasco and a team of four other researchers said their work showed direct effects of glyphosate that open "concerns about the clinical findings from human offspring in populations exposed to GBH [glyphosate-based herbicides] in agricultural fields." The findings in the lab are "compatible with the malformations observed in the offspring of women chronically exposed to GBH during pregnancy," Carrasco argued.[10] "I suspect the toxicity classification of glyphosate is too low," he said. "In some cases this can be a powerful poison."[11]

Carrasco went to great lengths to publicize his team's findings, presenting his findings at a press conference held at the 6th European Conference of GMO-Free Regions of the European Parliament in Brussels. He also coauthored a critical report on the sustainability of GMO soy that challenged fundamental industry assertions about the benefits of the technology and called Monsanto's dealings in Argentina "heavy-handed attempts to dominate global seed and glyphosate supplies." That September 2010 report included a litany of warnings:

The industry claims that glyphosate is safe for people and breaks down rapidly and harmlessly in the environment. But a large and growing body of scientific research challenges these claims, revealing serious health and environmental impacts. The adjuvants (added ingredients) in Roundup increase its toxicity. Harmful effects from glyphosate and Roundup are seen at lower levels than those used in agricultural spraying, corresponding to levels found in the environment. . . .

The cultivation of GM RR soy endangers human and animal health, increases herbicide use, damages the environment, reduces biodiversity, and has negative impacts on rural populations. The monopolistic control by agribusiness companies over GM RR soy technology and production endangers markets, compromises the economic viability of farming, and threatens food security.[12]

Not surprisingly, Monsanto challenged Carrasco's assertions and the credibility of his research. The company said his methodology was flawed and used unrealistic exposure scenarios. "Public health experts agree that Carrasco's experiments with frog and chicken embryos are not predictive of health effects in humans or wildlife," the company said in a posting on its website.[13] "Regulatory authorities and independent experts agree that glyphosate does not cause adverse reproductive effects in adult animals or birth defects in offspring of these adults exposed to glyphosate, even at doses far higher than relevant environmental or occupational exposure."[14]

At the time, Carrasco was generally well regarded. Not only was he a neuroscientist at the University of Buenos Aires with expertise in embryonic development, but he was also head of the research department at the Ministry of Defense and principal investigator and past president of the National Scientific and Technical Research Council (CONICET), a highly respected Argentine research institute.

In part because of the high regard for Carrasco's work and the troubling nature of his findings, a group of environmental lawyers filed a petition with the Supreme Court of Argentina seeking a ban on glyphosate, and the Ministry of Defense announced a ban on glyphosate use on some of its land that was used for agricultural production. Activists and others who had long been convinced that agrochemicals were to blame for health problems in their communities rallied around the scientist.

But Carrasco also quickly found himself with multiple enemies after he went public with his work on glyphosate. The Chamber of Agricultural Health and Fertilizers (CASAFE), which represents Monsanto and the other agrochemical industry interests in Argentina, sent representatives to visit Carrasco's laboratory looking for documents related to his research, the scientist told the press. The scientist also reported receiving anonymous threatening phone calls. And he and a group of activists were reportedly physically attacked at an August 2010 gathering in the small farming town of La Leonesa, where Carrasco was scheduled to speak about his glyphosate study. Press accounts said Carrasco and a colleague locked themselves inside a car as an angry mob yelled threats and beat on the vehicle. The minister of science, technology and productive innovation, Lino Barañao, considered a chief government supporter of Monsanto, discounted Carrasco's findings and criticized him for sharing his results with news outlets before they were published in the peer-reviewed scientific journal *Chemical Research in Toxicology* a year and a half later.[15]

When Carrasco died from an extended illness at the age of sixty-seven in May 2014, he was described in the press as one of Monsanto's "most difficult public relations problems."[16]

Javier Souza, a regional coordinator for the Pesticide Action Network in Latin America, said that despite the questions raised about glyphosate by Carrasco and others, the power and prestige of the agrochemical companies combined to keep the chemical in common use. "The concerns are very great," he said. "There is increasing evidence on the possible effect of glyphosate on health, yet both business and family producers are increasingly using it."[17]

A group of fifteen Argentine farmers and their eight children tried to take their concerns about Roundup-related health problems to court in February 2012, suing Monsanto and other companies over allegations that the farmers' use of Roundup and other glyphosate-based herbicides in growing tobacco on their family farms had caused birth defects in their children. The farmers would mix and spray the pesticides from applicators they carried on their backs, and they often were accompanied in the fields by their spouses. Although at the time they thought they were handling one of the safest chemicals available in agriculture, they now believe their exposure to the weed killer caused their children to suffer a range of problems, including spina bifida. Not only were they exposed when they applied the herbicides, but the chemical also contaminated the farmers' nontobacco crops, water wells, and streams, they claimed. "Monsanto has marketed glyphosate as posing little or no risk to human or environmental health when in fact Monsanto knew or had reason to know that aforementioned herbicide is a reproductive toxin, teratogenic, genotoxic and otherwise harmful," the farmers claimed. They said they were encouraged by Monsanto to use large amounts of the weed killer, "frequently and in quantities beyond what would be necessary for effective weed control. Defendants did this purely to increase profit."[18]

The farmers tried to pursue their lawsuit in the United States, but a Delaware judge dismissed the suit in November 2015, saying the claims were too vague and giving the farmers an option to amend their complaints against Monsanto.[19] The farmers then refiled in January 2016 and have continued to press their claims.

The United States government has been no idle observer of the angst in Argentina. Indeed, the U.S. Embassy in Buenos Aires kept a close eye on the developments, reporting updates to the U.S. secretary of state, the U.S. Department of Agriculture (USDA), the U.S. Environmental Protection Agency (EPA), and others as Argentina wrestled with what, if anything, to do about the pesticide concerns. Cables obtained and released by WikiLeaks provide some hints of the level of the embassy's interest and action and demonstrate in many cases that U.S. officials were eager to promote and sustain the use of glyphosate. In one cable dated May 7, 2009, shortly after Carrasco's research came to light, the embassy wrote that the "campaign against the use of glyphosate" appeared to be driven "more by local politics than health concerns." The embassy called Carrasco's findings "unverified" and said that while both the Ministry of Defense and the Ministry of Health were expressing concerns about glyphosate, the National Service of Health and Agrifood Quality (SENASA) and the Ministry of Science, Technology and Productive Innovation were defending glyphosate's use. The embassy said Monsanto had the largest share of the glyphosate market in Argentina, estimated at 40 percent, making the company "the most prominent and vulnerable victim" of the "attacks" on glyphosate. The embassy said it was providing information to SENASA as it built a case for continued glyphosate use in Argentina.[20]

The embassy concluded that it was unlikely the country would implement a ban on glyphosate because the economic impact could be substantial, with soybean production estimated to drop by 20 percent without glyphosate to help control weeds. The cable concluded with a note reassuring U.S. agencies that Argentine support for biotech seeds and for glyphosate was unlikely to be disrupted. Too much money was at stake:

> Argentina has long been an ally of the United States with respect to biotechnology promotion in various international negotiations, and Roundup Ready biotech soybeans are Argentina's most important export crop. Post contacts within the Secretariat of Agriculture assure us that Argentina will continue to support biotechnology . . . and none of our contacts believe that the GOA will go so far as to ban the use of glyphosate, or Roundup Ready soybeans.[21]

The United States had good reason to support the notion that glyphosate use in South America was safe. Not only were sales of glyphosate worth billions of dollars to U.S.-based Monsanto, but also, starting in the year 2000, glyphosate had been a key tool in a program promoted by the U.S. government to fight the South American drug trade. U.S. officials believed glyphosate, sprayed either from the ground or from the air, was an effective way to wipe out crops of opium poppy, used to make heroin, and coca crops used for cocaine. Colombia was a key target for the mission. Members of Congress worried that "Plan Colombia" could jeopardize the health of people living in sprayed regions, as well as damage the environment, but other U.S. leaders saw the program as an effective way to remove a lucrative source of income from Colombian drug groups. The U.S. Department of State reassured those who were worried about glyphosate, reporting that the EPA had found that "there is no evidence of significant human health or environmental risks from the spraying" in Colombia.[22] Under the program, the United States provided technical and scientific advice, the glyphosate herbicide, fuel, spray aircraft, and a limited number of escort helicopters. The actual spray aircraft were piloted by either U.S. citizens, Colombians, or third-country national contractors. The U.S. government hoped for the same arrangement in Peru, but government officials there would not agree.

The aerial spraying in Colombia also did not sit well with officials in neighboring Ecuador, who claimed glyphosate drifted across the border the countries share, harming hundreds of people who were exposed to the pesticide. An Ecuadorian commission issued a report in 2007 that said the herbicide mixture used in the Colombia spraying was highly toxic and was causing health and environmental damage. The country asked for limits on spraying close to its border and for financial compensation for the people impacted.

The U.S. Embassy publicly appeared to stay clear of the dispute between the two countries, but privately embassy personnel expressed their "belief that glyphosate is safe" and encouraged the government in Ecuador to consider that other factors might be to blame for the health and environmental problems it was attributing to glyphosate.[23] Ecuador did not back down, however, and in 2013, Colombia agreed to pay $15 million to settle a lawsuit filed by Ecuador for human and economic damage caused by the Colombian spraying of glyphosate.[24]

Colombia suspended the glyphosate fumigations in 2015 because of the mounting evidence of health and environmental dangers, including fears the aerial spraying might be putting people at risk for cancer. The decision came after IARC's classification that glyphosate was a probable human carcinogen. U.S. officials pressed the Colombian government to continue the program, and by early 2017 the government had resumed the use of glyphosate, using workers to spray the chemical on the ground by hand rather than from the air.

~

The diplomatic interest in the glyphosate debates in Argentina, Colombia, and Ecuador are only a few examples of a much broader program under which U.S. taxpayers have been footing the bill for overseas lob-bying of the products developed by Monsanto and other seed and agro-chemical makers. There are hundreds of diplomatic cables between the U.S. State Department and embassies in more than one hundred coun-tries that show State Department officials as active promoters of the types of GMO soy, corn, and cotton that took over Argentine agricul-ture. Expanded use of those glyphosate-tolerant crops meant more use of glyphosate and higher sales for companies producing the chemical. The cables show that U.S. officials often worked to quash any public criticism of the technology, the chemicals, and the companies, such as Monsanto, selling the products. The cables also show that U.S. diplo-mats supported Monsanto's work abroad even after the company was charged with bribing an Indonesian official and violating the Foreign Corrupt Practices Act in 2005. Monsanto ultimately paid a $1.5 million fine in that case.[25]

One 2009 cable showed that the U.S. Embassy in Spain sought "high-level U.S. government intervention" at the "urgent requests" of Mon-santo to combat biotech crop opponents there. The cables also reveal that State Department officials instructed embassies to "troubleshoot problematic legislation" related to biotech crops, and to "encourag[e] the development and commercialization of ag-biotech products." The State Department also produced pamphlets promoting GMOs in Slove-nia, sent pro-GMO industry DVDs to high schools in Hong Kong, and helped bring foreign officials and media from seventeen countries to the United States to promote biotech agriculture.[26]

The details contained in the cables deepened suspicions that the U.S. government does more to promote global acceptance of biotech crops than to protect the public from harm. "I believe that our government is more interested in pushing ag biotech interests than looking objectively at independent science data that shows the potential harmful effects," said Pamm Larry, a U.S. activist who has called for more scrutiny of GMOs and glyphosate. "Why is it that our tax dollars are being used to force countries and their citizens to use and consume products they don't want from an industry that's poisoning the planet?"[27]

Another South American country caught up in controversy over glyphosate is Paraguay, which borders Argentina to the north. As in Argentina, Paraguay's landscape has been transformed as it became a leading supplier of GMO glyphosate-tolerant soy. Aerial spraying of farm fields with glyphosate and other chemicals has forced many people from their villages and raised health concerns like those seen in Argentina. People living near the farm fields have complained that their rivers have become contaminated with the pesticides used on the soybeans, and they have reported rising rates of birth defects in their children. Farmers have found it hard to grow anything but the glyphosate-tolerant soy because other crops die if they come into contact with the herbicide, which drifts from field to field.[28]

For Judy Hatcher, who served as coleader of the international Pesticide Action Network and as executive director of the North American arm of the organization for five years, until June 2017, the U.S. government's work to promote pesticide products enriches powerful corporations such as Monsanto at the expense of poor and vulnerable populations. "Time and time again, global pesticide corporations have exerted far too much influence over government policy," said Hatcher. "Family farmers around the world are demanding the right to good health, not more exposure to hazardous pesticides, and are looking for greater control over their lives, seeds, farms, and livelihoods, not locked into Monsanto's model."[29]

CHAPTER 9

Uproar in Europe

To some, the suggestion seemed more than a little unusual: members of the European Parliament, who were deep into a debate over the risks and rewards of glyphosate in the spring of 2016, should take a close look inside themselves before voting on whether or not to ban the controversial pesticide—literally. The Green Party, whose platform backs environmentally sustainable policies, pushed the idea of a "pee test," as the press called it, in hopes of demonstrating the pervasiveness of the chemical's reach and underscoring the very real personal implication of the political decisions being debated. Though some dismissed the idea as a political stunt—a "pissing contest"—48 of the 751 parliament members agreed to submit their urine for scrutiny by researchers at Bio-Check, a diagnostic laboratory located in the German city of Leipzig, Saxony. They handed over their samples in April and awaited the results, though not necessarily with eagerness.

At the time, the battle brewing over glyphosate was at a fevered pitch. The European Commission was preparing to approve a new fifteen-year authorization for glyphosate before the June 2016 expiration of the current license. But several European Union (EU) members were mounting fierce opposition to the plan as people across Europe protested reau-thorization. The French National League Against Cancer—La Ligue nationale contre le cancer—started a petition drive seeking a ban, and a Belgian organization of medical and public health professionals known as the Health and Environment Alliance (HEAL) also weighed in to demand a ban, urging European cancer societies to take a similar stand. Supporters of a ban were worried not only about ties the chemical might have to cancer but also about reported associations with birth defects, Parkinson's disease, and other ailments, as well as damage to the environment.

In response, the European Parliament passed a resolution suggesting that glyphosate not be approved for any longer than seven years and not be used at all in public places such as parks and playgrounds. The reso-lution cited concerns about cancer and endocrine disruption and said that the practice of spraying glyphosate on crops shortly before harvest to ripen them was unacceptable because it increased human exposure. The members of the European Parliament, who are commonly referred to simply as MEPs, called on the European Commission to invoke the precautionary principle before making a final decision on whether or not to keep glyphosate products on the market.[1] The idea of a precau-tionary principle took root in the 1980s in Germany, taking on global significance when included in a 1992 declaration made as part of the United Nations Conference on Environment and Development. The precautionary principle states that "where there are threats of serious or irreversible damage, lack of full scientific certainty shall not be used as a reason for postponing cost-effective measures to prevent environmental degradation."[2]

The political divide would grow even wider as the two bodies, which act as parts of the legislative branch for the twenty-eight countries that make up the EU, wrestled over concerns about the weed killer. Those who stepped up to speak out against continued glyphosate use cited the cancer classification made by the International Agency for Research on Cancer (IARC) and said the evidence of health risks was undeniable, far outweighing any benefits that made the chemical popular with many European farmers. Even though genetically modified crops are cultivated on only a tiny fraction of European farmland—primarily a small amount of GMO corn acreage in Spain—Roundup herbicide and other glyphosate weed killers have been a mainstay on conventional, nonorganic farms for decades, mainly because they were considered so much safer than other herbicides and because they worked so well.

In fact, while glyphosate was beloved by European farmers, the GMO crops developed to be used with glyphosate were another matter. Europeans never embraced the new high-tech tinkering with plant DNA. Wariness was so widespread that several countries banned any planting of them, including Austria, Poland, Hungary, Greece, and Germany. And shortly after they were introduced in the United States, European nations also tried to block any importing of GMO crops and products because of fears that the crops could be unsafe for people and the environment.

The United States spent years railing against Europe's reluctance to embrace GMOs. In 2003, U.S. officials brought a complaint with the World Trade Organization arguing that the European communities were violating international trade rules by effectively implementing a moratorium on imports of the specialty crops. The ban translated to substantial monetary losses for U.S. interests, of course, as American farmers were the largest producers of GMO crops, and U.S.-based Monsanto Company was the prime GMO developer. The U.S. Department of State asserted that as of 2002, lost sales of GMO corn and soy products amounted to at least $300 million.[3]

President George W. Bush took the complaint even further, declaring that the losses went beyond financial concerns and into the humanitarian realm. The Europeans who were thumbing their noses at the modern scientific magic of genetically engineered crops were actually contributing to starvation in Africa, he said. "Our partners in Europe . . . have blocked all new bio-crops because of unfounded, unscientific fears. This has caused many African nations to avoid investing in bio-technologies for fear that their products will be shut out of European markets," Bush said in a 2003 speech. "European governments should join—not hinder—the great cause of ending hunger in Africa."[4] The World Trade Organization ultimately agreed with the United States, and with Canada and Argentina, which raised similar complaints; the EU was ordered by world trade authorities to lift the ban.

With all the sparring over GMOs, worries about glyphosate were mostly sidelined for many years. A handful of outlier scientists and environmentalists kept tabs on the spread of the chemical, but few others paid attention. French scientist Gilles-Eric Séralini stirred global controversy with his findings that GMOs and glyphosate caused a range of health problems in rats, but for the most part many scientists toiled away on obscure research studies that got little to no attention until the mounting evidence of troubling ties to cancer and other illnesses became impossible to ignore. By the spring of 2016, when the MEPs submitted their own urine for glyphosate testing, worries about the weed killer had matched or surpassed the fears associated with GMOs. The links to cancer, as confirmed by IARC's review of several different research studies, made for more risk than many Europeans were willing to accept. Polls showed that two-thirds of Europeans supported a ban on glyphosate, including 75 percent of Italians, 60 percent of the French, and 56 percent of Britons.

Testing for glyphosate in urine, foods, and beverages was fairly widespread in Europe by that time, but interest had been growing for years as people wondered how much, if any, of the weed killer was making its way into their bodies. In 2012, Séralini and six other French scientists undertook a study aimed at measuring levels of glyphosate in farmers' urine. The scientists examined a farm family in which two of the family's three children had been born with birth defects. The farmer routinely used a hand sprayer to treat portions of his three fields and a tractor for others. The children were rarely in the fields. The scientists collected the farmer's urine for twenty-four hours the day before he sprayed and for two days after and found that "glyphosate was easily detected in the father's urine." There were also detectable levels of glyphosate in the urine of one of the farmer's three children, even though the family lived about a mile away from the field and the child did not help in the weed killer application. The scientists speculated that the child's exposure could be due to prolonged contact with his father, but the farmer thought this was "inconceivable," given the distance between their home and the fields.[5]

As it turns out, glyphosate doesn't show up only in the urine of farmers. A survey commissioned in 2013 by the advocacy group Friends of the Earth Europe found that people in eighteen countries across the continent had traces of glyphosate in their urine. Just how the chemical was making its way into people's bodies wasn't certain, but tests were also finding glyphosate residues in many types of foods, particularly bread made from wheat that had been sprayed with glyphosate shortly before harvest.

In Britain, the slogan "Not in Our Bread" became a rallying cry when the Soil Association, the country's leading organic certification organization, said that glyphosate residues had been detected in close to one-third of all samples of British bread and that glyphosate had been found to be a regular contaminant of bread products in routine tests by independent food safety experts. For whole grain products, the residue contamination was much higher, seen in almost two-thirds of the bread products. "If glyphosate ends up in bread it's impossible for people to avoid it," said Peter Melchett, policy director of the Soil Association.[6]

So it was perhaps little surprise, then, when the results of the MEPs' urine testing were announced in May 2016: every single parliament member who participated had tested positive for glyphosate. And, making matters worse, the pesticide was present at levels far higher than some expected. The laboratory said the average rate of glyphosate found in the MEPs' urine was 1.7 micrograms per liter, an amount that is roughly seventeen times the permitted level of glyphosate in European drinking water. The lowest level found among the group was 0.17 nanogram per milliliter (ng/ml), almost double the safe level, the Green Party said when it announced the results.

Jean Lambert, a member of the European Parliament's Agriculture Committee, described the results as "frightening." Her personal test results showed a glyphosate level of 0.67 ng/ml. "It is genuinely frightening that glyphosate is everywhere in our everyday lives," Lambert said. "These test results show that no matter where we live, what we eat, or our age we cannot escape exposure to this toxic substance. With glyphosate widely used in cities, in urban parks and public spaces, on streets and pavements, the European Commission must bow to public pressure and put the safety of people and the environment ahead of the profits of chemical industry giants."[7]

Green Party members announced the results publicly, using the social media hashtag #MEPee and the slogan "Let's Keep Pee Glyphosate Free." MEP Marc Tarabella told the local press, "The results of this milestone research should force the public and manufacturers alike to acknowledge that the omnipresence of a potentially carcinogenic and suspect substance, such as glyphosate, constitutes a phenomenal problem."[8]

The findings added to similar study results published a month earlier after the Heinrich Böll Foundation, which describes its mission in part as "defending the freedom of individuals against excessive state and economic power," looked at samples of urine from more than 2,000 people living in Germany. That research found levels of the herbicide in 99.6

percent of participants and found that roughly 75 percent of the people who gave samples had five times the amount of glyphosate in their urine than was legally allowed in drinking water. Children, particularly those raised on farms, had the most significant levels, the study found.[9]

The German Environment Agency, known as Umwelt Bundesamt (UBA) in its home country, also has looked at the glyphosate issue, conducting an analysis of urine in students over more than a decade. The results showed the presence of the weed killer in roughly 40 percent of students sampled in 2015, up from roughly 10 percent in 2001, with spikes as high as almost 60 percent in 2012 and 2013.[10] The UBA's president, Maria Krautzberger, said the signs that glyphosate is so pervasive that it commonly passes through children and adults, rural and city dwellers alike, should trigger more safety research and a cautionary approach to its use and regulation.[11]

But Germany's Federal Institute for Risk Assessment, known to Germans as the Bundesinstitut für Risikobewertung (BfR), had a different response. The BfR discounted the significance of glyphosate in urine, saying that the chemical is excreted out of the body rapidly and is not at all harmful. In other words, having a little of the pesticide in one's "pee" was nothing to worry about. "In our opinion, these very low levels are to be expected, since glyphosate is an approved active substance contained in plant protection products, meaning that residues could be expected to be ingested with the food and hence excreted," the BfR's president, Professor Andreas Hensel, said after the Heinrich Böll Foundation's study results were released. The BfR claimed the study had "major flaws," including what the BfR said was a perceived lack of proper handling of the samples. And the group said that while the levels may seem high, when calculated in the context of how much would be consumed, it was far less than the acceptable daily intake (ADI) set by regulators. "No adverse health effects are to be expected from glyphosate residues ingested with food," the agency said.[12]

The BfR also maintains that glyphosate does not cause cancer. Its own assessments show that "according to current scientific knowledge, no carcinogenic risk is to be expected if the substance is used correctly and in line with its intended purpose," the BfR states on its website.[13]

Confused? Determining who is right and who is wrong when it comes to glyphosate has been just as difficult in Europe as it has been in the United States. Activists say there is a simple explanation: Just as in the United States, the companies that sell glyphosate have wielded influence with a heavy hand. And just as the U.S. Environmental Protection Agency (EPA) relies heavily on the industry's own studies for its safety determinations, so too do regulators in Europe.

Take the BfR, for example. The BfR operates as a "scientifically independent institution" within the portfolio of the Federal Ministry of Food and Agriculture (BMEL) in Germany, but questions about just how independent the institution really is would come to cloud its work on glyphosate. The BfR's job is to advise the government on questions of food, chemical, and product safety, and it was a key advisor to the European Food Safety Authority (EFSA) when the agency reviewed glyphosate ahead of its expiration in 2016 and the bid for reauthorization. Not only did the European Commission want EFSA's recommendation about whether or not glyphosate should remain on the market, but also EU member states were relying on the agency to help them address safety questions about glyphosate products used in their territories.

After the World Health Organization's IARC team of cancer scientists classified glyphosate as a probable human carcinogen in March 2015, the European Commission asked EFSA to give special consideration to those findings—to see if there really were cancer risks Europeans might need to be protected from. And EFSA turned to the BfR to help analyze IARC's work.

The BfR did its advisory job thoroughly, drafting a detailed report that provided the basis for EFSA to declare in November 2015 that

IARC was flat out wrong about glyphosate's ties to cancer. In fact, EFSA claimed, evidence showed that glyphosate was actually "unlikely to pose a carcinogenic hazard to humans." EFSA said it had looked at more information than IARC had, and it was so satisfied with the chemical's safety that it also advised raising the allowed amount of glyphosate residue in food, saying the ADI level should nearly double, from 0.3 milligram per kilogram (mg/kg) of body weight per day to 0.5 mg/kg/day.

And those urine tests? EFSA has reassuring words for anyone worried about what the weed killer might be doing to their bodies. The safety agency said that absorbed glyphosate is "poorly metabolised, widely distributed in the body . . . and is rapidly eliminated; showing no potential for bioaccumulation."[14] Jose Tarazona, head of EFSA's Pesticides Unit, said the conclusions followed "an exhaustive process—a full assessment that has taken into account a wealth of new studies and data."[15] What Tarazona did not say publicly was that EFSA's conclusions also came after the EPA's Jess Rowland, the official who Monsanto considered a reliable friend inside the agency, engaged in a teleconference with EFSA in September 2015, explaining why EFSA should reject a 2001 study that found a causal link between glyphosate exposure and tumors in Swiss albino mice. Records show the agency did exactly that.[16] It was that same month, in an e-mail dated September 3, 2015, that Monsanto's regulatory affairs leader, Dan Jenkins, wrote to colleagues how "useful" Rowland could be in "ongoing glyphosate defense."[17] EFSA said there was no industry attempt to improperly influence its assessment of glyphosate, but skeptics were not satisfied.

Monsanto, which stood to lose an estimated $100 million in sales if its license for glyphosate were not renewed in Europe, applauded the BfR's and EFSA's safety findings.

EFSA's conclusions, which came eight months after IARC said glyphosate was probably carcinogenic, provided much-needed ammunition for Monsanto and the other chemical companies as they headed into 2016, when glyphosate's registration would expire and the European Commission would be deciding about reauthorization.

The BfR and EFSA were so enthusiastic about glyphosate safety that they sent representatives to the United States in December 2016 to appear before the EPA's Scientific Advisory Panel on glyphosate and tell the group how safe both agencies found glyphosate to be. The EPA said it did not request that either EFSA or the BfR appear; instead, the agencies themselves said they decided to travel across the ocean to make their arguments.

So where did the BfR get the data for its report to EFSA? From none other than the Glyphosate Task Force, a consortium of chemical companies, including Monsanto, that had joined forces with the stated goal of winning renewal of glyphosate's registration in Europe.[18] The BfR acknowledged as much, saying the health evaluation prepared for glyphosate was based on publications and other "relevant information" submitted by the industry consortium as well as on older studies that were part of previous EU evaluations. The BfR also claimed that because so many studies were submitted, it was unable to look at them all in detail, so it relied on the industry consortium "descriptions and assessments" of the studies rather than going through each independently.

The revelation outraged some who saw the circumstances as a blatant example of industry interests taking precedence over protection of public safety. Greenpeace called EFSA's report a "whitewash" that relied heavily on unpublished studies commissioned by glyphosate producers while dismissing published peer-reviewed evidence that glyphosate causes cancer. "EFSA has defied the world's most authoritative cancer agency in order to please corporations like Monsanto," said Greenpeace EU's food policy director, Franziska Achterberg.[19] Other environmental and consumer groups also complained that the findings lacked independent scrutiny.

"We know that Monsanto and other companies provided their own assessment of the scientific evidence, much of it industry-sponsored unpublished studies, and then handed that pig off to Germany for some lipstick," said Jennifer Sass, a senior scientist with the Natural Resources Defense Council. That "industry-dominated" finding of unlikely cancer ties should be discounted because its credibility was too compromised, she said.[20]

A group of ninety-six scientists, including some members of IARC's panel, penned a critical letter to the EU's commissioner for health and food safety, a man named Vytenis Andriukaitis, imploring the European Commission to "disregard the flawed EFSA finding on glyphosate . . . and to call for a transparent, open and credible review of the scientific literature." The scientists, who hailed from several countries, including New Zealand, Australia, Germany, Switzerland, France, Italy, Russia, and the United States, said that IARC's decision was the truly credible one because it relied on "open and transparent procedures by independent scientists who completed thorough conflict-of-interest statements and were not affiliated or financially supported in any way by the chemical manufacturing industry." In contrast, the scientists wrote, the BfR's and EFSA's work "is not credible because it is not supported by the evidence and it was not reached in an open and transparent manner."

Among other problems, the scientists said, it appeared that EFSA was disregarding significant positive trend findings in animal studies that showed links between glyphosate and tumors in mice and rats, that it was differing from standard scientific practices, and that it was ignoring "unequivocal" evidence of the carcinogenicity of glyphosate in laboratory animals. And particularly troubling to the scientists was the lack of information about unpublished studies the government agencies seemed to be relying on.[21] The criticisms of the European regulators were nearly identical to those lobbed at the EPA. "Due to the potential public health implications of this extensively used pesticide it is essential that all scientific evidence be freely available, reviewed openly in an objective manner, and that financial support, conflicts of interest and affiliations of authors be fully disclosed," the scientists wrote.[22]

One of the signatories, Xaver Baur, senior professor at the Charité Institute of Occupational Medicine in Berlin, made a detailed presentation to the European Parliament stressing the research tying glyphosate to rising rates of non-Hodgkin lymphoma and describing the various other cancers and disorders his clinic sees in farmers and agricultural workers exposed to glyphosate and other pesticides. He said there are potential parallels between the glyphosate situation and that of asbestos, which chemical industry players defended for decades despite what became overwhelming evidence of asbestos's ties to lung cancer. "Precaution is strongly recommended," he told the gathering, saying the cumulative impacts of exposure through food and the environment are currently unknown. Glyphosate and its formulations represent "a new potentially hazardous internal load to the human body and the health risk is incalculable at present."[23]

Such widespread skepticism led to demands from consumer advocates and MEPs for EFSA to release the actual unpublished studies provided by Monsanto and other industry players to show glyphosate was not cancer-causing. The hope was that by looking at the studies themselves, rather than the industry-aided interpretation, outsiders could determine whether or not EFSA's assessment was accurate. A group called Corporate Europe Observatory, a watchdog organization that tracks corporate lobbying in the EU, was among those seeking the studies. The group said that clinical trial data for new medicines is routinely made public to enable scientific scrutiny, and the same should be done for agrochemicals such as glyphosate. Similar requests had been made over the years to other global regulatory authorities, which commonly cited business confidentiality restrictions imposed by the industry in refusing to make the data public. The studies were trade secrets, according to Monsanto, even though they were used in multiple countries to seek approvals for products sold to, and used by, the public.

A chink was notched into that argument's armor in 2013 when the Court of Justice of the European Union ruled on a legal complaint filed by environmental groups that challenged the secrecy over glyphosate. The court ordered that any document containing information about emissions into the environment needed to be released to the public.

The ruling made it difficult for EFSA to keep the data secret, but the agency still showed reluctance to full disclosure. E-mail communications obtained through public access requests in Europe showed that EFSA went to Monsanto and the other pesticide companies who owned the relevant studies to seek permission to release certain documents, including a feeding study of mice that had been dosed with glyphosate. As was expected, the companies objected to the disclosures. Monsanto was adamantly opposed to letting members of the public view its research results and analysis, arguing that its work represented intellectual property and such information could aid competitors by supplying them with "key commercial information." The company underlined some of its objections in a letter to EFSA. The following are a few excerpts:

> Monsanto hereby formally objects to the disclosure of the entirety of the Study. . . .

> Our objections are also grounded by legitimate economic interests protected by the confidentiality.

> The Study represents a material investment in time and money for Monsanto. . . .

> . . . Should EFSA still consider granting access to the document to the third party, Monsanto would insist on making The Study available to the third party in a closed data room, without any

possibility to make copies, reproduction or communication of the information and under logistical conditions to be agreed with Monsanto. . . .

Prior to the third party viewing The Study, Monsanto would request an opportunity to sanitise The Study. . . .[24]

Despite Monsanto's objections, the political pressure on EFSA would eventually force the agency to release the raw data, sending the genotoxicity and carcinogenicity studies it used in its assessment to a group of MEPs who had submitted a formal request for the information. Before sharing it, however, EFSA blacked out numerous sections, saying it had to balance the public's "right to know" with its obligations to protect "commercially sensitive information."[25]

Industry influence also colored a report from another group that weighed in to support glyphosate. This group of eighteen scientists, officially known as the Joint FAO/WHO Meeting on Pesticide Residues (JMPR), made their analysis as part of a program administered by the Food and Agriculture Organization of the United Nations (FAO) and the World Health Organization (WHO). They were generally considered to be experts in their fields and independent of industry influence. But the group that was called to meet in Geneva, Switzerland, in May 2016 to review IARC's work on glyphosate did not exactly meet the latter standard. The JMPR group included several scientists who were members of, or who worked for, the chemical industry. There was little surprise when the JMPR scientists declared that, like EFSA's, their review determined that glyphosate was probably not carcinogenic to humans. But there was plenty of condemnation. "There is a clear conflict of interest here if the review of the safety of glyphosate is carried out by scientists that directly get money from industry," said Vito Buonsante, an attorney with the nonprofit environmental law group ClientEarth.[26]

The complaints about the chemical and the secretive studies behind the regulatory approval were so unrelenting in early 2016 that the European Commission, which was planning a vote on glyphosate's reauthorization for March, found itself facing what *The Guardian* newspaper dubbed a "mutiny."[27] The French Agency for Food, Environmental and Occupational Health & Safety (ANSES) was among those leading the revolt, issuing a report in February that contradicted EFSA, saying that its own assessment of the research showed glyphosate could "arguably" be classified as "suspected of being carcinogenic to humans."[28] ANSES said there were serious concerns not just about glyphosate but also about the other chemicals, the co-formulants, used along with it in herbicide products. The French agency said it was launching a new review of glyphosate and polyethoxylated tallow amine (POEA) combinations, and it called on the European Chemicals Agency (ECHA) in Helsinki, Finland, to step in to review the research on glyphosate. Government representatives from the Netherlands also called for any relicensing to be put on hold until completion of ECHA's evaluation. Italy and Sweden joined forces with France and the Netherlands in a show of opposition that was sufficient to convince the European Commission to postpone the March vote until May. But opposition only grew stronger, and that vote was again postponed when Germany said it would abstain from voting because of a divide within its ruling coalition. The dissent left the European Commission without a majority needed to either relicense or ban the chemical.

By the end of June, just days before the authorization for glyphosate was to expire, the European Commission said it would postpone any decision on glyphosate for at least a year, granting an eighteen-month extension for glyphosate products while authorities awaited the results of the new evaluation. During the extension, glyphosate use should be minimized on playgrounds and in parks, the EU member states decided.

Amid the uproar, the Germany-based chemical conglomerate Bayer AG made a takeover bid for Monsanto, an overture that eventually would lead to a $66 billion proposed deal, which is still pending as of this writing. And angry Europeans organized a citizens' initiative seeking a ban on glyphosate.

By early 2017, European uncertainty regarding glyphosate safety had only grown deeper. ECHA announced in March that after reviewing "extensive scientific data," it had concluded glyphosate should not be classified as a carcinogen, and it said it took into consideration both published studies and the original reports of studies conducted by industry.[29]

That failed to reassure many MEPs, however, and in April 2017 thirty of them penned a letter to the president of the European Commission, Jean-Claude Juncker, questioning the trustworthiness of the data relied on by regulators to vouch for glyphosate safety. They cited the internal Monsanto documents revealed through the U.S. cancer lawsuits as cause for alarm. The group was particularly upset about Monsanto communications that discussed ghostwriting research and the fact that at least one study that regulators trusted appeared to have been authored by a scientist who Monsanto had recruited and paid specifically to attach added credibility to the work.

The MEPs also pointed to internal company documents that surfaced in the court case showing the company wrestling with how to handle genotoxicity concerns about glyphosate and Roundup. The corporate records showed that in the late 1990s the company was very worried about scientific research indicating that Roundup was genotoxic, including a mouse study by Italian scientists published in 1997 that saw DNA damage in the livers and kidneys of animals treated with the weed killer. "Despite the many positive aspects of glyphosate use, there are some data that indicate its technical formulation, Roundup, is a potential toxic agent. The formulated commercial product, Roundup, seems to be rather more toxic than the parent compound," the scientists concluded.[30]

To try to beat back growing concerns about its herbicide, in 1999 Monsanto brought in a genotoxicity expert named James Parry—an authority in the field of mutagenicity in the United Kingdom—to lend his opinion. After reviewing both published studies on glyphosate and Monsanto's unpublished in-house studies, Parry did not deliver the resoundingly positive findings Monsanto had hoped for. Instead, he concluded that glyphosate showed at least some potential to be genotoxic, damaging to human health. Parry recommended that Monsanto undertake additional tests. But rather than follow Parry's advice, Monsanto executives declared they would not do such studies and discussed finding another expert to dig them out of a "genotoxic hole." Executives questioned whether Parry had "ever worked with industry before."[31]

In one internal e-mail, Monsanto scientist William Heydens wrote:

We want to find/develop someone who is comfortable with the genetox profile of glyphosate/Roundup and who can be influential with regulators and Scientific Outreach operations when genetox issues arise. My read is that Parry is not currently such a person, and it would take quite some time and $$$/studies to get him there.

Even if we think we can eventually bring Parry around closer to where we need him, we should be currently looking for a second/back-up genetox supporter. We have not made much progress and are currently very vulnerable in this area. We have time to fix that, but only if we make this a high priority now.[32]

As well, the documents revealed that for many years Monsanto employed a Belgian toxicology expert named Mark Martens to advise the Belgian government and the EU on pesticide registration issues and provide a "toxicology defence of Monsanto products in the EU." Monsanto would later recognize Martens for working to "protect Monsanto's bottom line" and for the development of "data to gain key EU scientific support that the reported genotoxicity of Roundup herbicide was due to secondary consequences unrelated to glyphosate, thereby preventing adverse effect on Roundup business."[33]

The revelations in the e-mails worried the MEPs enough that they urged Juncker to "fully investigate whether Monsanto has deliberately falsified studies on the safety of glyphosate" and to set up a "black list of the companies which use lies as a common policy." The MEPs also asked for a ban on undisclosed contacts between European Commission officials and any Monsanto lobbyists.[34] Juncker dismissed the MEPs' concerns and said there was no reason to question the regulatory assessments of safety. As of this writing, the European Commission was proposing to reauthorize glyphosate for ten years, even as critics argued that doubts about the chemical's safety should not be ignored.

~

In Italy, a country known for its wine and pasta, the battle over glyphosate, or *glifosato*, as the Italians call the chemical, is as passionate as it is political. Farmers such as Rolando Manfredini, who raises fodder for cattle and sheep in the mountainous Modena Apennines region, have seen worries about the herbicide steadily rising across Italy for years. Vineyard operators, fruit and vegetable growers, cereal grain producers, and ranchers have started casting a more wary eye on the weed killer. In a country renowned for both natural beauty and fresh, wholesome foods, growers fear that glyphosate residues are a shadow over both human health and the vitality of the soil and water.

"Farmers are very worried about the safety of this chemical," said Manfredini, who oversees food safety issues for Coldiretti, the country's main farmers' organization. Coldiretti, founded in 1944, counts among its members more than 1.5 million farmers and a number of Italian companies engaged in agriculture. "Italy has leadership in terms of food safety. Italian farmers are very concerned about its residues, for their health but also for consumers and the environment."[35]

Cancer statistics show that non-Hodgkin lymphoma, the type of cancer with the strongest link to glyphosate, is the eleventh most common cancer in Europe, with approximately 93,500 new cases diagnosed in 2012. And incidence rates of the cancer in men are higher in Italy than in all the rest of Europe.[36]

Italy's Ministry of Health placed several restrictions on the use of glyphosate in the late summer of 2016, banning it in areas frequented by the public, especially places where children or elderly people might gather. In addition to parks and gardens and areas around schools, the chemical was banned along roads and railways and in areas adjacent to health-care facilities. The Ministry of Health also said the preharvest use of glyphosate would not be allowed. Even though Canadian and U.S. farmers had made the practice common—on wheat, for instance, or on oats in Canada—spraying crops with glyphosate shortly before they are harvested was deemed too risky for consumers in Italy because of the residues that remain on finished foods. The package of restrictions marked one of the widest bans on both consumer and agricultural use of the controversial chemical.

Andrea Ferrante, a leader within the Italian organic farming movement and former head of the Italian Association for Organic Agriculture (Associazione Italiana per l'agricoltura biologica), said organic farming enthusiasts are encouraged to see the tide turning against glyphosate. Even many conventional farmers who have been using glyphosate are trying to move away from it, including winemakers in Tuscany, a region famed for production of top wines. "There is quite a movement giving evidence on how harmful glyphosate can be," Ferrante said. "We have so much scientific data, so much research about its cancer origin activity, that it's also easy for us to explain to the rest of the world why it is so harmful for the environment and human health."[37]

CHAPTER 10

When Weeds Don't Die, But Butterflies Do

History has shown that proving a specific chemical causes cancer is a long road that can leave countless lives in limbo for decades while the science is sorted out. But when it comes to the impact a certain chemical can have on the environment, often the evidence is easier to see. In fact, sometimes it is impossible to miss.

I encountered my first superweed in 2011 and was both impressed and a bit horrified by the stature and strength of the towering stalks. I had been hearing farmers complain about weed problems, but I didn't truly appreciate the magnitude of the concern until that hot August afternoon when a group of Kansas farmers gave me a tour of their troubles. These were no pesky annoyances that one could easily yank out by hand or kill with a quick dousing of herbicide. The weeds I saw were almost taller than I was. Once wiped out with a few shots of Roundup or other glyphosate product, many types of weeds by that time had become impervious to the pesticide. Thwarting ever-higher doses of the weed killer, they just kept on growing, sinking roots deep down into farm fields, stealing nutrients and moisture from corn, cotton, soy, or other crops a farmer might try to grow.

One of the worst to emerge has been a weed called Palmer amaranth, a particularly stout variety that can grow three inches per day and rob farmers of about two-thirds of their corn and soybean yields. The Palmer amaranth, part of a family known as pigweed, has developed resistance to many other types of herbicides as well, making it a significant threat to crop production. It can grow eight feet tall, with a stem so tough that it can damage farm machinery. Another rapidly spreading weed, known as water hemp, has similarly become a bane to farmers. Water hemp can grow an inch per day and stretch as tall as twelve feet. Each plant generates 250,000 seeds, or more, that can hide in the soil for as long as four years before emerging to ruin a farmer's production hopes. The weeds are much more than an annoyance; they spell real economic harm to farmers and others up the food chain.

The world has long dealt with resistance problems—the rise of anti-biotic resistance in medicine has become a global public health concern, making it difficult to treat illnesses and infections. Several different weeds have developed resistance to other herbicides over the decades. But the rise of glyphosate-resistant weeds happened with such speed and intensity after Monsanto Company's introduction of genetically engi-neered glyphosate-tolerant crops that many farmers and others in the agricultural community were caught by surprise.

"Monsanto told them that it would never happen, despite all the aca-demics trying to raise concerns about it," said agronomist Bill Johnson, a professor of weed science at Purdue University. "When the first cases of resistance popped up, Monsanto fought that tooth and nail. You had a huge industry pushback on the whole diagnosis."[1]

Before the introduction of the genetically modified crops, farmers had to carefully select and time the use of various herbicides to manage weeds without harming their crops. Many also frequently rotated the types of crops they planted from season to season and year to year, alternating corn with wheat, soy, oats, or other crops as a time-tested way to maintain the health of the soil and naturally reduce insect pests and weed development. A row crop such as corn tends to bring higher prices for farmers but is known for depleting the soil of needed nutrients, while legumes such as alfalfa and clover actually store nitrogen in their root systems, which then break down after harvest and help fertilize and restore soil health. They also are known to help the soil better absorb water. Cereals such as oats also have dense root systems that feed the soil organic matter. Sunflowers, sorghum, canola, mustard, and snap beans are among the crops that once were favored in the U.S. Heartland as players in healthy crop rotations. It's been accepted almost as agricultural gospel for generations—the more diverse the cropping system, the fewer problems overall, including weeds. That message began to get lost, however, as the number of small family farms in America declined, evolving into fewer but larger operations. Between 1935 and 2012, the number of U.S. farms fell from more than 6 million to roughly 2 million, though farming acreage remained fairly stable.[2]

The evolution saw farmers focus on growing fewer crops that produced higher profits. Diverse rotations that included three or four different crops were starting to become a thing of the past, and farmers were relying more on an array of chemicals to fight weeds even before the introduction of genetically engineered crops. Weed specialists such as Johnson would commonly write prescriptions for farmers, detailing for them exactly which herbicides to use, how much to use, and when to apply the various chemicals to their fields to tackle different types of weeds.

But when farmers were handed the magic of glyphosate-tolerant corn, soybeans, and other crops, the cautious prescriptive approach faded fast. Farmers didn't need multiple herbicides and didn't need to carefully time their use. They also didn't need to worry about rotation. Farmers could plant the same few GMO crops year after year, spray them all directly with glyphosate, and then sit back, relax, and tally up their projected profits. They still had to contend with the whims of Mother Nature and commodity markets, of course, but weeds were taken care of. When Monsanto's patent on glyphosate expired in 2000, prices fell as generics came to market, making it even more appealing for farmers to rely on glyphosate.

It was easy and effective, no doubt about it, but it also was a practice that prioritized short-term profits over long-term environmental sustainability. Many environmental scientists warned that the path was a dangerous one to follow, and they were proven right when, less than a decade into the advent of genetically engineered glyphosate-tolerant crops, farmers found themselves caught in a vicious cycle. As farmers used more glyphosate to kill the resistant weeds, the weeds became more resistant. And so on.

By 2010, researchers estimated that these superweeds infested close to 33 million U.S. farm acres.[3] The following year, in the summer of 2011, the federal government was so worried that representatives from the U.S. Environmental Protection Agency (EPA), the U.S. Department of Agriculture (USDA), and the Weed Science Society of America took a tour of the Midwest crop belt to see for themselves the impact of rising weed resistance. By 2013, researchers reported the problem had nearly doubled, with more than 61 million acres infested with glyphosate-resistant weeds. Researchers at Kansas State University, who were scrambling to assess the depth of the problem, found that even spraying weeds with up to four times the typical application of glyphosate failed to kill them. By 2014, agricultural experts were recommending that farmers resort to deep tillage to destroy the weeds, a practice that churns up the earth to remove weeds but can also lead to soil erosion, chemical runoff, and other environmental problems. And by 2016, more than 70 million acres were infested.

"Herbicide resistance can increase pretty rapidly, once you have a few resistant plants survive," said Dallas Peterson, a weed specialist and professor in the Department of Agronomy at Kansas State University, who has been tracking the resistance problem. "It can kind of explode on a farmer in a given field. The first year, there's a few scattered plants, but it's not too bad. The next year there's a few more, and by the third year, it's kind of a disaster if the farmer hasn't made any adjustments to his weed management program."

Peterson visits regularly with farmers to advise them on how best to tackle weeds. And he had been among those who warned many years ago that relying too much on glyphosate would bring problems. He's not happy to have been so right.

"To be honest with you, the effectiveness of Roundup kind of spoiled us," he said. "It was very easy. We got away from some good, sound weed management practices and just relied on another glyphosate application. Eventually it caught up with us."[4]

Researchers first started documenting a significant rise in glyphosate-resistant weeds around 2001 in the United States and have shown the plague spreading with each passing year. Glyphosate-resistant weeds are also documented in Argentina, Brazil, Paraguay, Canada, Mexico, and several European countries—almost anywhere glyphosate has been used, weeds have been fighting back. But the bulk of the problems with resistant weeds have been seen in the United States, where glyphosate-tolerant crops have been widely used. Resistant Palmer amaranth spread from California to North Carolina, alongside more than a dozen other resistant weed types. Farmers in key crop-producing states such as Iowa, Illinois, Missouri, Georgia, and Mississippi have become unhappily accustomed to seeing their fields invaded by the almost unstoppable weeds.[5]

The southeastern United States has been hardest hit, with more than 90 percent of cotton and soybean fields infested. Cotton farmers in the South have been forced to hire crews to walk through fields and attack each weed by hand, obviously an expensive approach. In Georgia alone, farmers have been spending roughly $15 million per year on hand-weeding rows of cotton, and their annual herbicide costs have jumped from $25 million per year to approximately $100 million per year as they pour on more chemicals to try to combat the weeds.[6] Overall, agriculture experts estimated that by 2016, U.S. farmers were losing an estimated $2 billion annually as a result of added costs and diminished yields.

The problems are quite personal for Illinois wheat, corn, and soybean grower Dean Campbell, a fifth-generation farmer working land that has been in his family's hands for 170 years. Campbell was one of the first farmers in rural southern Illinois to start using Roundup Ready soybeans when they came on the market in 1996. He remembers neighbors coming to marvel at his fields covered in gorgeous "clean" beans—not a weed in sight. "We had swallowed the pill as far as soybeans go. Plant them and spray them with Roundup and go on," he recalls. But within just about five years, Campbell started noticing that not all the weeds in his fields would die after he applied a typical treatment of glyphosate. "I knew right away there was something wrong," he said. Within a decade of using the glyphosate on his soybean fields, Campbell was fighting "monster" weeds with every tool he could think of. "You hang them, you stab them, you poison them, you shoot them, you do everything you can to stop them," the sixty-four-year-old farmer said, only half in jest. "We're running out of tools."[7]

He remembers with particular bitterness one season that brought a "beautiful" crop of beans but also weeds that sprouted and grew so quickly that they towered over the baby bean plants before Campbell could intervene. Glyphosate would not kill the weeds because of the resistance, and he couldn't spray any other herbicides because those would have also killed the beans. Campbell had no choice but to plow the field and start over.

Campbell now tries a variety of strategies: he's rotating wheat with his beans, making sure he does a thorough "burn down" of his fields before planting—meaning he coats the soil with weed killer a few weeks before planting—and he scours his fields daily as the new crops start to grow, catching and killing or pulling weeds while they are still small. If they get taller than an inch or two, "there is no stopping them," Campbell says of the weeds.

Part of what makes it all so frustrating for agricultural scientists is that there were plenty of predictions of the problems to come when Monsanto introduced its glyphosate-tolerant crops in the mid-1990s. Glyphosate had been on the market for twenty years before the GMOs were rolled out, and no significant problems with glyphosate-resistant weeds were noted. But environmental scientists knew that the system Monsanto was promoting was a perfect incubator for resistance. They were proven right when more than a dozen weed species quickly evolved to resist the herbicide. Weed scientists from academic institutions around the country rang the alarm bell as long ago as 2004, forming a group called the National Glyphosate Stewardship Forum (NGSF) to try to warn farmers about the risks they faced as they cast aside traditional cropping practices for reliance on glyphosate. The group reached out to commodity organizations as well as the EPA and conservation groups to alert them to the impending calamity and to urge more restrained use of glyphosate. But many farmers were unconvinced. If they had not yet dealt with the superweeds in their own fields, they had little incentive to alter their practices. Monsanto balked as well, rejecting calls for regulatory or other limits and downplaying the problem. The company assured farmers that some weeds reported as resistant really weren't and that strategies for dealing with the weeds should be developed on a case-by-case basis and not be imposed on farmers. "Regulations are not necessary. Once regulations start, they do not stop," the company said in a presentation made to the first meeting of the stewardship forum. The meeting, conveniently, was held in a hotel in St. Louis, Missouri, not far from Monsanto's headquarters.[8]

Three years later, the frustrated consortium of weed scientists met again in St. Louis to renew their plea to be heard and to discuss why the warnings they had issued in 2004 fell on deaf ears. The group's report did not use the words "we told you so," but the message was clear: "We expected that grower and staff leaders from the commodity organizations would express concerns about potential resistance, request further information, and ultimately support or propose additional steps for action. However, the participants were uniformly unconvinced that glyphosate resistance in weeds was a significant threat at that time. The participants reached consensus that any glyphosate stewardship efforts should be voluntary and without governmental intervention." Since then, the task force said, "numerous additional cases of glyphosate-resistant weed populations have evolved and several weed species with glyphosate-resistant populations have become difficult and expensive to manage. . . . It is time for action."[9]

Bryan Young, a weed scientist who grew up on a farm in Michigan taking prize sugar beets to the county fair, understood why farmers ignored the warnings. Glyphosate made everything so simple. Rotating crops and varying herbicides was complicated, and farmers preferred the easy answer. "We were kind of spinning our wheels telling growers about resistant management," Young said of the period from the mid-1990s to the mid-2000s. "At that time there wasn't a lot of evidence that this could be a problem."

The EPA was of no help. Young, who now works at Purdue University as a professor of botany and plant pathology, was among a group of worried scientists who met with agency officials, asking them to help alert growers and possibly require more sustainable practices in order to keep glyphosate effective and protect both the environment and long-term productivity on American farms. But the EPA also turned a deaf ear to the warnings in those early years, Young recalled. "I think they've changed their minds now. But it could be too little, too late."[10]

One of the most troubling impacts of the glyphosate-resistant weed problem has been a resurgence in use of other herbicides, many of which are much more directly toxic than glyphosate. Farmer Campbell has resumed use of paraquat, for instance, the deadly chemical linked to Parkinson's disease, which is known to be so dangerous that a skull and crossbones symbol is shown on labels for paraquat products. Inhaling or ingesting it causes almost certain death. He can't spray it on his crops or they will die, but it works well on bare ground before crops are planted. Later, he'll spray the same fields with glyphosate.

The use of other chemicals is also on the rise because the chemical industry's answer to the weed resistance problem has been simple— more chemicals, mixed together. Farmers are being more careful to "clean" their fields before planting with herbicides, and they are mixing glyphosate with other weed-killing chemicals in the spray tanks they drive into their fields.

And now a whole new generation of herbicide-tolerant crops, designed to be used with new herbicide mixtures, is coming to the market. Just as with Monsanto's Roundup Ready system, farmers can spray the new weed-killing chemical combinations directly on their new genetically engineered crops. And just as in the Roundup Ready system, glyphosate remains key.

One of the most prominent of the new herbicide products combines glyphosate with 2,4-D, the sixty-five-year-old chemical that became infamous as an ingredient in the Agent Orange defoliant used by the United States during the Vietnam War. Dow AgroSciences raised the ire of environmentalists and health advocates alike when it asked for the EPA's approval for the product it calls Enlist Duo. According to USDA estimates, by 2020 the new glyphosate and 2,4-D herbicide is likely to lead to a 700 percent rise in the use of 2,4-D, which the

International Agency for Research on Cancer (IARC) classifies as "possibly" carcinogenic to humans. Some scientists say that 2,4-D is a suspected endocrine disruptor that has been linked to reproductive harm and that children are particularly susceptible to its effects. Dow's own research has shown harmful impacts, but the EPA has agreed to allow more than forty times more 2,4-D into the American diet than was previously permitted, all in an effort to fight glyphosate-resistant weeds.[11]

Another highly touted new herbicide combination, glyphosate and dicamba, also spells trouble, according to assessments by some scientists and environmental groups. Monsanto's new Roundup Ready Xtend system is expected to push dicamba use from less than 1 million pounds annually to more than 25 million pounds annually. Farmers are encouraged to plant GMO crops that are tolerant of both dicamba and glyphosate so they can be sprayed directly with both to kill weeds. While many farmers have welcomed the new options, dicamba exposure has been associated with lung and colon cancer and birth defects and, like glyphosate, with non-Hodgkin lymphoma. And a rise in dicamba use is also expected to be harmful to birds and mammals, including some endangered and fragile species.[12] Several farm groups and environmental organizations filed a federal lawsuit in January 2017 alleging the EPA violated its charge to protect people and the environment by approving the new use of dicamba along with glyphosate pesticides.

The growing use of dicamba and 2,4-D may also be bad news for farmers because the herbicides are generally known to have "high volatility," meaning they tend to drift easily into neighboring fields, where they can kill crops not genetically designed to be sprayed. Documented crop losses from just such drift have already been seen in many states. The Missouri Department of Agriculture tallied more than one hundred drift damage complaints in 2016, for instance. Farmers there alleged that dicamba sprayed by other farmers wafted into more than 41,000 acres of Missouri soybeans, peaches, tomatoes, rice, cotton, peas, watermelon, and more, killing or severely injuring the crops. The issue often pits farmer against neighboring farmer, and it is so serious that law enforcement authorities cited drift damage as a motive in the murder of a fifty-five-year-old Arkansas farmer who was shot to death during an argument over apparent herbicide damage to his crops. The farmer had filed a complaint with Arkansas officials about the crop damage before he was killed, and he had spoken publicly about his anger over the issue. A farm manager who was working land just across the border, in southern Missouri, was arrested and charged with first-degree murder in the case. The two men had arranged a meeting to discuss the drift problems when the shooting occurred, in October 2016, according to law enforcement.[13]

Monsanto and the other agrochemical companies have worked to reduce the volatility of the herbicide products they are introducing to combat glyphosate resistance. And the EPA is placing some restrictions on use to try to reduce the risk of drift damage. Both the companies and the regulators argue that more and better chemicals are the best answers to fighting the failures in the field. But critics say this perpetual chemical race against Mother Nature amounts to an ever-faster and more dangerous pesticide treadmill that loads more and more chemicals onto an already ravaged landscape. And, they say, it won't work. Combining old chemicals into new mixtures used on top of herbicide-tolerant crops may provide a short-term fix, but the strategy has no hope of success over the long term. Weed resistance will only increase with the increased chemical use.

"Monsanto's Roundup Ready crops created an environmental disaster by causing infestation of tens of millions of acres of farmland with herbicide-resistant weeds and spurring an enormous increase in pesticide use," said Earthjustice attorney Paul Achitoff, who has sued the EPA over these issues. "Planting more GE crops and dousing them with more noxious chemicals isn't the answer. The Environmental Protection

Agency should be protecting health and the environment, not Monsanto's profits."[14]

The current model simply isn't sustainable, says Stanley Culpepper, a professor at the University of Georgia who specializes in crop and soil science. Georgia, the United States' second-largest cotton-producing state, has been hit harder than many others by weed resistance; the problem impacts most of the state's 1.1 million acres planted to cotton. Culpepper, who grew up on a cotton plantation, works closely with cotton farmers across the state to try to come up with the best ways to beat back the weeds, and he has tracked the rising costs and challenge for growers. More than 90 percent of the state's farmers now hand-weed their cotton fields, he said. The need for reforms is immediate—and obvious, in his view. And while pesticides are an important tool, they can't be the only tool.

"My opinion as a scientist, if our goal is to feed the world, we cannot do it today without pesticides," said Culpepper. "But we have to treat them with respect. Anytime we can use them more economically and in a more environmentally friendly way, that's what we want to do. We're not sustainable if all we're going to do is go out and spray stuff."[15]

Back in Indiana, Purdue's Young said it may be a message farmers don't want to hear, but it is an inescapable reality: "When you talk about managing herbicide resistance by using more herbicides, it's just counterproductive. Right now it may seem like the best option because it's the most available and effective. But in the long term, is it sustainable? No."[16]

Jumping off the pesticide treadmill in favor of more sustainable solutions is easier said than done, especially when the corporations developing and selling the chemicals keep pressing for more. It's understandable; every gallon sold adds to corporate revenues, after all. But just as they've done in other dicey debates involving their products, the chemical industry players have turned to some friendly—and financially linked—academics to help convince regulators and the public to embrace their new herbicide and herbicide-tolerant crop combinations.

One key ally has been David Shaw, vice president for research and economic development at Mississippi State University and past president of the Weed Science Society of America (WSSA). Shaw has had significant influence in helping shape policy on weed resistance in the United States, chairing a task force that developed a USDA report that made recommendations on how to address the problem, and counseling the EPA on the same. As many other agricultural experts were warning of the dangers of new herbicide-crop combinations, Monsanto could count on Shaw's help to convince the USDA to green-light the company's new Xtend herbicide-tolerant soybeans and cottonseed. Monsanto had supported Shaw with research grants totaling at least $880,000 since 2002, and the company seemed quite comfortable asking him to step in on its behalf. Monsanto specifically wanted Shaw to refute arguments made by environmental and consumer advocates that the company's new products would increase potentially harmful herbicide use.[17] As Monsanto knows, when the message comes from an expert who appears to be independent of industry, it usually carries more weight.

Monsanto executives asked for Shaw's help on multiple occasions in 2012 and 2013, asking him to write letters of support to regulators—conveniently providing specific prose and policy points that Shaw should include—and to engage in other activities, such as participating in a government-held meeting on the controversy. E-mails obtained between Monsanto executives and Shaw showed that the company was feeling pressured by the chorus of opposition to the company's new herbicide-tolerant cropping system.

"In a way this boils down to a numbers game which means we can't just sit back and let the opposition dominate the conversation," Monsanto's in-house weed expert, John Soteres, wrote to Shaw in June 2013, asking him to call in to a USDA meeting on the company's dicamba products. Soteres helpfully suggested what Shaw should say, and Shaw agreed to call in. Soteres wrote to Shaw after the call: "I think I owe you a really good steak for this one."[18]

Dow AgroSciences also relied on Shaw to help it win over regulators for its new 2,4-D and glyphosate herbicide and cropping system. Just as Monsanto did, Dow asked Shaw to reach out to regulators in support of its products, even offering suggestions for how Shaw should word his message. In one communication, a Dow scientist named Larry Walton reminded Shaw that the company was "providing some very good scholarship funding" for Mississippi State University graduate and undergraduate students.[19]

Both Monsanto and Dow ultimately received government approvals for their new products, victories that are expected to bring well over $1 billion in added revenues to the companies. Monsanto's win was also a win for consumers, according to the company. "Weeds represent a key pest to agriculture operations around the world and limit crops of much-needed nutrients, sunlight and access to available water resources," Robb Fraley, Monsanto's chief technology officer, said in touting the regulatory approval. "We're excited to provide additional tools that can help improve efficiencies on farm and support farmers in bringing more food to harvest for consumers."[20]

For farmer Campbell, the challenges ahead will soon be someone else's to manage. He expects to be the last in his family to run the 2,800-acre farm. His son declined to follow in his father's footsteps, instead pursuing a career as an electrical engineer, and his daughter became an attorney; neither has a desire to build a future in the small rural community of Coulterville, Illinois, population 945, that borders the family farm. Campbell doesn't blame them a bit, he says. Making a living as a farmer has never been easy, and the evolution of agriculture is always challenging. His generation's intensive use of agrochemicals may not be the best choice for the future. He hopes that the next phase of technology and tools for farmers will support, rather than thwart, sustainability.

"Who can fathom what we'll be doing sixty to seventy years from now?," he said. "I don't consider myself an environmentalist, but I am a realist. I have a grandson and two granddaughters. . . . I want them to all have somewhere to live and something to eat. The environment . . . it's fragile. We don't want to destroy it."[21]

~

While weed resistance has drawn intense scrutiny because of the immediate economic impacts, the widespread use of glyphosate has created many other less visible, but potentially just as costly, environmental problems. And one of the most poignant is the demise of the iconic monarch butterfly, a migratory creature that typically winters in central Mexico or coastal California and then moves to summer breeding grounds in the northern United States and Canada. The fluttering of the monarch's distinctive black, orange, and white–patterned wings as it flits from flower to flower has long been a familiar sight in gardens, fields, and meadows. But the population has been in steep decline over the past few decades, dropping by more than 80 percent between the mid-1990s and 2016. Since 1990, about 970 million have vanished, according to the federal government. Researchers project that the monarch could disappear almost entirely by 2036.[22]

The losses mean much more than extinction of a beloved North American species; they translate to a direct impact on the health of the environment. Monarchs, like their butterfly brethren, are among a group of insects and animals that pollinate an array of living plants. Bees are considered probably the most important, as they pollinate key food crops. But butterflies are also significant, particularly for pollination of native wildflowers, as they pick up pollen and carry it to other plants in their search for sweet nectar.

And why should anyone care too much about wildflowers? Other than adding color to the landscape, flowering plants produce breathable oxygen, they help purify water and prevent erosion by means of root systems that hold soil in place, and they return moisture to the atmosphere. The delicate environmental interplay is one we tamper with at our own peril.

Both bee and monarch populations have been in decline, and while scientists have tied bee deaths to a class of agricultural insecticides known as neonicotinoids, research shows that the demise of the monarch is linked directly to heavy use of glyphosate. The proliferation of the herbicide that came with genetically engineered glyphosate-tolerant crops has obliterated native plants that are key food sources for young monarchs, primarily a plant known as milkweed. Monarch butterflies depend on milkweed to provide places to lay their eggs and offer nourishment for the caterpillars that hatch. But in Iowa, for example, cropland lost 98.7 percent of its milkweed from 1999 to 2012, and it is estimated that in the same time span there was a 64 percent overall decline in milkweed in the Midwest. Glyphosate, either sprayed directly or drifting on the breeze, has sharply reduced both the abundance and diversity of milkweed and other plants that provide nectar for butterflies. In the past twenty years, monarchs have lost an estimated 165 million acres of habitat—an area close to the size of Texas.

In a petition to the U.S. Department of the Interior, which has responsibility for upholding protections within the Endangered Species Act, a consortium of environmental and food groups explained the problem this way:

> A primary threat to the monarch is the drastic loss of milkweed caused by increased and later-season use of the herbicide glyphosate in conjunction with widespread planting of genetically-engineered, herbicide-resistant corn and soybeans in the Corn Belt region of the United States and to planting of genetically-engineered cotton. . . .

Glyphosate used in conjunction with Roundup Ready crops has nearly eliminated milkweed from cropland throughout the monarch's vital Midwest breeding range.[23]

Other threats endanger the monarch's survival, including shifting weather patterns attributable to climate change; conditions that are too hot or too cold at critical times in monarch development can kill both young and adult monarchs. Development of millions of acres of natural habitat has also played a role. But without their essential food supply, the monarchs are doomed regardless of other factors, scientists say.

To try to save the monarch, a partnership of U.S. state and federal agencies and environmental groups launched the Monarch Joint Venture in 2014. As part of that effort, the U.S. Fish and Wildlife Service started encouraging people to plant milkweed—in flower boxes, in parks, along roadsides, anywhere and everywhere. The agency itself said it would plant milkweed in refuges and other areas it controls, with a goal of creating 200,000 acres of habitat for the monarch along the butterfly's north–south migration route.[24] To motivate the public, the joint venture also launched multiple social media campaigns, including a monarch Facebook page and Twitter account. The group sells T-shirts and water bottles emblazoned with butterfly images, asking members of the public to become monarch "ambassadors."

Even the White House, under President Barack Obama, got involved, announcing a "national strategy" in 2015 to save the bees and butterflies. One goal: restoring populations to at least historic averages of about 225 million monarchs overwintering in Mexico by 2020. The White House said at least 7 million acres would need to be restored as friendly habitat for the bees and butterflies, and it called on all federal agencies, which control more than 41 million acres across the United States, to incorporate "pollinator-friendly" practices in landscaping and construction projects on federal land.[25] As part of the president's national strategy, the EPA said it would evaluate a number of actions that could be taken to protect monarch butterflies, including restrictions on how glyphosate and other agrochemicals are handled. But as of this writing, little has been done on that front.

Monsanto has not shied away from the monarch issue; instead it has acknowledged that a reduction in milkweed plants in farmland across the Midwest is among factors contributing to the butterfly losses and that glyphosate has been linked to those losses. The company has sought out discussions with the EPA regarding glyphosate and the monarch, saying it wants to be part of a solution:

> As research continues, the pressing question for all of us is: what can we do to help? We're talking with scientists about what might be done to help the monarchs rebound. And we're eager to join efforts to help rebuild monarch habitat along the migration path by joining with conservationists, agronomists, weed scientists, crop associations and farmers to look at ways to increase milkweed populations on the agricultural landscape.
>
> There's no reason agriculture can't coexist with natural wonders like monarch butterflies and their annual migration.[26]

Monsanto pledged at least $3.6 million and 100,000 milkweed plants to aid in monarch restoration efforts. Still, the company's push for the use of glyphosate in combination with other herbicides to address weed resistance, critics say, will only add to the threat to the monarch.

～

Potentially even more worrisome than the superweeds and the declining monarch butterfly population is the subtle change glyphosate appears to be having on the soil, the lifeblood for plant life, including the fruits and vegetables we eat and the crops that feed our cattle, chickens, and hogs.

Robert Kremer, a research microbiologist who served in the USDA's Agricultural Research Service for thirty-three years before retiring in 2014, stumbled across unsettling changes in the soil several years ago while conducting his government research in a laboratory at the University of Missouri. Born and raised in a farming family, Kremer knew, through both his upbringing and his education, that maintaining a healthy balance of the microorganisms living in the soil is critical to healthy crop production. When the balance is off, crops are more susceptible to disease and can lack needed nutrients. Farmers might need to use more chemicals to try to aid the ailing crops, or watch them wither away.

Kremer's work to document how soil properties, plant growth, and soil microorganisms were influenced by agricultural practices was done quite literally in the shadow of Monsanto—his office was located near a Monsanto-funded building on campus that housed Monsanto Auditorium. The university is located only about one hundred miles west of Monsanto's St. Louis–area headquarters, and the company's influence in the state and at the university was well known. Early in Kremer's career there, he was part of a team of researchers who received roughly $500,000 in Monsanto grant money. At that time, in the late 1990s, there was little controversy in soil science. Kremer was well regarded by the USDA and well-liked by the student scientists he mentored at the university. While his study of the soil was interesting to other scientists, rarely did it get much attention from the general public.

But with the rise of genetically modified crops and the surge in the use of glyphosate to go with them, Kremer's research findings took a disturbing turn. He started seeing that the roots of Roundup Ready crops that had been sprayed with glyphosate became ravaged, swarmed with harmful fungi. While the aboveground part of the crop appeared to be tolerating the herbicide treatment well, the roots showed that was not necessarily the case. The soil changes left plants more vulnerable to disease, interfered with the absorption of beneficial nutrients, and could leave the harvested grain with a reduced nutritional composition, in Kremer's view. It became apparent to him over time that repeated use of glyphosate was damaging farm fields given over to glyphosate-tolerant cropping systems, even if the effects were largely invisible to the farmer. He also found that glyphosate, released into the ground through the roots, can persist in the soil for one to two years, depending upon several variables, including the type of soil. That meant farmers wanting to rotate or plant conventional crops that weren't glyphosate tolerant risked crop damage from the chemical lingering in the soil. Kremer published his ongoing research in scientific journals, hoping to alert regulators and others to the concerns.

"We might be setting up a huge problem," Kremer said. This is supposed to be a wonderful tool for the farmer . . . but in many situations, it may actually be a detriment. We have glyphosate released into the soil which appears to be affecting root growth and root-associated microbes."[27]

Monsanto has always maintained that glyphosate does nothing to harm the delicate and highly complex soil microbial communities that are critical to maintaining the health and quality of soil. "Soil microbes and microbially influenced processes are not adversely impacted by field-rate applications of glyphosate," the company asserts.[28]

After Kremer started to speak out about his findings, he found they weren't necessarily welcomed by the agricultural and regulatory community—even within his own agency, the USDA. He had been allowed to talk freely to members of the press in the past, but starting in the late 1990s, as GMOs and glyphosate use were surging in popularity, the ability to speak freely as a government scientist faded. "There was this whole atmosphere that we didn't want to offend anyone in the ag industry," Kremer recalled. "Well, I offended some people."

Kremer was told that if he spoke about his research findings involving glyphosate or GMO crops, any presentations he made must be approved not only by his local USDA supervisor but also by staff at national head-quarters. "There was, I don't want to say censorship, but quite a bit of editing that went on," Kremer said.

Kremer knew how influential Monsanto could be; when he and a colleague were awarded the $500,000 Monsanto grant a decade earlier, the company had "wanted to completely control the research," he said. But he was still surprised when several USDA colleagues, one whom he considered a very close friend, authored a report that he felt dismissed much from his years of research.

The study was led by botanist Stephen O. Duke, the same USDA scientist who in 2008 declared glyphosate an "environmentally benign" resource and asserted that there was no conclusive documentation of harmful glyphosate impacts on or within the soil.[29] Duke told me he does not see his research as contradicting Kremer, but Monsanto has touted the Duke report to discount Kremer's findings. It's noteworthy that Monsanto and Duke have had a long and close affiliation through an agrochemical industry–sponsored organization called AGRO. Duke has served as a member of the AGRO executive board for several years and chaired the group in 2014. There is no financial arrangement or benefit associated with serving as chair or fellow to AGRO, Duke said. Still, the group, a division of the American Chemical Society, is funded by Monsanto, DuPont, Dow, Syngenta, and other corporate chemical powerhouses. Having government scientists so closely affiliated with corporate interests can jeopardize the independence of their research, critics say.

For his part, Kremer is glad to be retired and free of the political pressures. He spends his time teaching a few classes at the university and making presentations about his research to agricultural groups around the country. Soil is a "limited, nonrenewable resource," Kremer now warns farmers, advising them that careful stewardship is needed to protect it. He suggests that farmers reduce their glyphosate use, use cover crops, and rotate herbicide-tolerant crops with non-GMO crops. It's a hard sell, Kremer knows.

Even his family's farm, located in the Missouri foothills of the Ozarks, grows glyphosate-tolerant corn and soybeans. The cropland is rented to a cousin, while Kremer's brother raises free-range hogs that are fed non-GMO grain and are raised without use of antibiotics, reflecting a growing divergence in farming practices. The family is working on a plan to transition to non-GMO corn and soybeans to reduce, and possibly eliminate, glyphosate on the farm fields.

Kremer has not been alone in his concerns about glyphosate's impacts on soil and plant health. Similar concerns have been raised by agronomist Michael McNeill, who consults with farmers in and around Algona, Iowa, right in the heart of corn country. The corn crop is so important to the area that a local newspaper produced an eight-page special section in January 2016 titled "Salute to Corn." Corn, after all, is king in Iowa. The state typically produces more than 2 billion bushels per year and not only is the top U.S. corn-growing state but also usually grows about three times the amount grown in all of Mexico. Most Iowa corn is glyphosate tolerant, which means applications of a lot of glyphosate. It's been fertile ground for research by McNeill, who holds a doctorate in quantitative genetics and plant pathology from Iowa State University and has been a crop consultant for more than three decades.

As farmers have applied more and more glyphosate over the years, McNeill has seen what he believes is nothing less than man-made destruction of soil health. "When you spray glyphosate on a plant, it's like giving it AIDS," he has said. His own observations dovetail with Kremer's findings, and he also has tried to sound the alarm, warning that overuse of glyphosate makes crops more susceptible to disease. He sees glyphosate as similar to DDT in its trajectory—hailed initially as a boon for society, only to be found later to carry hidden dangers.[30]

Some agricultural experts believe overuse of glyphosate has played a role in the devastation of Florida's citrus crop—a phenomenon that has been unfolding unbeknownst to most consumers, but one that has been all too real for the farmers who have been struggling to save their orange groves from the crippling disease referred to as "citrus greening." The disease also affects lemons, grapefruits, and other citrus crops, but it is the plague's impact on the orange industry that has left the state reeling. Florida produces more oranges than any other U.S. state, and citrus production is worth an estimated $9 billion to the state's economy. But since the disease showed up, around 2005, orange trees have been dying off faster than new ones can be planted, and yields from trees that survive have been in decline in recent years. Growers largely blame bacteria that take hold in the roots for causing their trees to produce green, disfigured, and bitter fruit, the "citrus greening" effect, which some scientists refer to by its Chinese name, huanglongbing. The bacteria choke off nutrient flow to the tree, sickening and ultimately killing it. As many as 69 million citrus trees in nearly all the state's groves have been infected, and orange production has slipped to the lowest levels in decades, costing the industry billions of dollars in lost sales. Florida's orange production was a robust 242 million boxes in the 2003–2004 season before the disease set in, but it was only 81 million boxes in the 2015–2016 season. Total U.S. orange production in 2015–2016 was down to an estimated 5.4 million tons, largely because of citrus greening, which has spread to Texas and California—a drop of 57 percent over 2004, according to the USDA.[31] The declines are not only harmful for orange producers; they also mean higher orange juice prices for consumers and—if not reversed—the scarcity of a staple of American breakfast.

The problem is so dire that the federal government has spent well over $200 million to try to come up with ways to combat the disease. Among the solutions explored is genetic engineering; research has been under way for the past few years to develop genetically modified orange trees that could resist the disease. The industry has expressed concern that consumers might reject GMO oranges and orange juice. But many researchers say it's the best way to address the problem.

Other researchers say they have a much simpler answer—stop using glyphosate. Farmers don't spray glyphosate directly on their orange trees, of course, but they commonly use it around the base of the trees and in the rows between trees to kill weeds that compete for moisture and nutrients in the soil. Over time, glyphosate's harmful effects on the micronutrients in the soil, seen by Kremer in soybean fields and by McNeill in cornfields, have left orange groves unable to fight off disease, some scientists believe.

"Extended use of glyphosate can significantly increase the severity of various diseases," Purdue University scientist Gurmukh Johal wrote in a research paper published in 2009. "Ignoring potential non-target detrimental side effects of any chemical, especially used as heavily as glyphosate, may have dire consequences for agriculture such as rendering soils infertile, crops non-productive, and plants less nutritious."[32] Along with glyphosate, many growers mix in additional herbicides to tackle weeds, loading up the soil with toxins.

"They don't understand it's the practices that are causing the problems," said crop consultant Frank Dean, who has been pushing the USDA and Florida farmers to consider soil deficiencies as part of the problem.[33] Dean is a product manager at a Texas company that sells agricultural fertilizers and microbial-based agricultural treatments to aid plant health, including a product that Dean says can help restore the health of orange groves. Many say his claims about soil problems being connected to citrus greening are nothing more than an effort to sell more products. But his work has the support of at least one USDA scientist. Craig Ramsey, who works with the agency's Animal and Plant Health Inspection Service, has collaborated with Dean on trying to alert government officials and farmers about the soil problems related to glyphosate. "All animals and humans, if we have a compromised immune system, we can be more susceptible to illness or diseases. Plants are the same; they have a great immune system to be able to fight off disease, but they have to have the nutrients to be healthy," Ramsey said.[34]

The USDA has given short shrift to theories that glyphosate damages the soil. Still, the questions aren't going away. Iowa farmer Mike Verhoef learned the hard way after he started growing glyphosate-tolerant corn and soybeans on his 300-acre farm in the tiny community of Sanborn. He made sure to rotate the corn and beans with oats to try to help replenish and balance the nutrients in his soil. Still, he noticed that the soil started to change, becoming harder to work, and his oat production dropped precipitously. He eventually gave up on the glyphosate-tolerant crops and went back to conventional crops that could not be doused directly with glyphosate. "I'm not turning back," he said, "because I haven't seen anything that is going to change my mind about glyphosate."[35]

CHAPTER 11

Under the Influence

So where, one might ask, are the regulators? The U.S. Environmental Protection Agency (EPA) has top authority over glyphosate, just as it does for other chemicals, but the agency has repeatedly discounted concerns about the chemical's impact on people and the environment, relying on a helping hand from industry to guide its actions. We've seen the cozy relationship between Monsanto Company and regulators play out over and over. We saw it in the 1980s, when EPA officials reversed the findings of agency scientists who considered glyphosate to be a possible human carcinogen; when the EPA followed Monsanto's lead in ignoring concerns about weed resistance until it was too late; when the EPA raised the legal tolerance levels for the amount of glyphosate that could be in our food even as cancer concerns were growing; and again in 2016, when the EPA rearranged its Scientific Advisory Panel on glyphosate at industry demand. And, of course, Monsanto's connections to, and appearance of assistance from, the EPA's top cancer assessment official, Jess Rowland, speak volumes about the strength of corporate influence within the agency.

U.S. congressman Ted Lieu, in early 2017, called for the U.S. Department of Justice to probe any EPA misconduct with its review of glyphosate. "We need to find out if Monsanto or the Environmental Protection Agency misled the public," he said.[1] Four other members of the U.S. House of Representatives called for a congressional investigation of the EPA's actions, saying, "We owe it to the American public to make sure . . . that the health of our children is prioritized over the profits of chemical companies."[2]

Lieu also asked the EPA's Office of Inspector General (OIG) to investigate any potential collusion between Monsanto and Rowland to bias the agency's review of glyphosate, and in May of 2017 the OIG agreed. Investigators were looking into several agency glyphosate review-related matters, the Inspector General's office said. That followed notification in 2016 by the OIG that it was probing the EPA's handling of glyphosate weed resistance problems.[3]

But the EPA is hardly unique in its attitude toward glyphosate or its willingness to bend to corporate pressure. The U.S. Department of Agriculture (USDA) and the U.S. Food and Drug Administration (FDA) not only green-lighted but promoted the use of glyphosate-tolerant crops, all while repeatedly refusing to scrutinize what levels of residue the chemical has been leaving in our food. Even when the FDA did start—and then suspend—limited efforts to look for glyphosate residues in food in 2016, the agency tried to keep negative findings a secret, telling scientists not to answer questions from the press and public about their work. It certainly could not have hurt to have former Monsanto vice president Michael Taylor sitting at the helm of the FDA as deputy commissioner for foods. Taylor has been held up as an example of the "revolving door" between industry and regulators, working at the FDA in the 1970s before joining a law firm that represented Monsanto, then going back to the FDA, and then joining the USDA just prior to a four-year stint at Monsanto. He returned to the FDA in 2009.[4] Such volleying of individuals between industry and government has become common.

Indeed, all three agencies have a history of close connections not just to Monsanto but to the chemical industry as a whole, and all have come under harsh criticism by consumer advocates for appearing to prioritize corporate pursuits over the health and well-being of private individuals.

But it is also true that each agency has deep wells of scientific knowledge and expertise—dedicated specialists who toil as mostly anonymous public servants with no industry affiliation. I've talked with several myself over the years, including during the writing of this book, and have found many good people—talented and honest soldiers hoping to use their skills to serve the public good. But I have also found time and again that many fear speaking "on the record," being quoted by name, regarding the work they are doing. They are proud of their research, but they also know that if their findings don't dovetail with powerful corporate interests, there can be hell to pay. They say research findings are sometimes suppressed, censored, and altered if not perceived as industry friendly. It often boils down to a simple calculation. As one senior government scientist who was worried about glyphosate but fearful of talking publicly told me, "I need to keep my paycheck."

One former EPA research scientist, retired now for over a decade, has no hesitation in expressing his view. "These pesticide companies, they claim they are helping to feed the world. That is a bunch of garbage," said Ramon Seidler, a microbiologist and retired senior scientist and former team leader for the EPA's biosafety program. "They are just helping themselves sell more products, and those products are deadly. Glyphosate should be banned entirely, but the industry has brainwashed folks in key decision-making positions in Washington. That's the way the system works."

Seidler says the fact that regulators rely on the chemical companies to run the safety testing of their own products is a fundamental problem but one that is deeply ingrained in the system. "Everybody knows that is not right. Industry should not be running the tests," he said.

Seidler, who has been listed by the International Biographical Centre of Cambridge, England, as one of the 2,000 outstanding world scientists of the twentieth century, and who was a recipient of the EPA's Bronze Medal for research service, says research indicating that glyphosate is an endocrine disruptor warrants strong and independent regulatory oversight. It angers him that the agency where he spent seventeen years doesn't do more to protect people, particularly children.[5]

A look inside these regulatory bodies shows decades of internal struggles to balance the interests of the public with those of powerful corporations that pressure agencies to protect profitable products such as glyphosate. This dynamic is seen in the handling of issues ranging from formaldehyde to arsenic and clean air to climate change.

If and when the EPA does move to ban a chemical from the market, it's often only after long-drawn-out battles with environmental and public health organizations and overwhelming scientific evidence of harm. Dow's battle to keep chlorpyrifos on the market despite evidence of detrimental effects on brain development in babies and young children is but one example. Insiders say that when millions, or billions, of dollars are at stake, political winds blow hard and sometimes public safety is sacrificed. Key pressure comes from members of Congress, who are recipients of the often-lucrative campaign donations doled out by industry and who control the budgets for these agencies. Elected officials not only control the purse strings but also can interfere through legislation or investigations. And, of course, the agencies themselves are run by political appointees who answer to the White House. It all adds up to a system of oversight that is often ineffectual, overwhelmed, and corrupt.

Attempts have been made to divorce politics from the regulation of toxic chemicals. When President Barack Obama took office in 2009 he pledged as much, promising in his inaugural address to restore science to "its rightful place" and citing the need for a more "watchful eye" over market forces. Obama's appointee as EPA administrator, a chemical engineer named Lisa Jackson, made the commitment directly to EPA employees after taking the reins: "The President believes that when EPA addresses scientific issues, it should rely on the expert judgment of the Agency's career scientists and independent advisors. When scientific judgments are suppressed, misrepresented or distorted by political agendas, Americans can lose faith in their government to provide strong public health and environmental protection," Jackson wrote in a January 2009 internal EPA memo to employees.

Jackson, whose career included sixteen years as an EPA staffer prior to her appointment, singled out regulation of chemicals as one of many areas in need of reform: "It is clear that we are not doing an adequate job of assessing and managing the risks of chemicals in consumer products, the workplace and the environment. It is now time to revise and strengthen EPA's chemicals management and risk assessment programs," she wrote in that memo.[6]

Under Obama, the EPA, the USDA, and other agencies were ordered to establish policies to protect scientific integrity and outlaw politically driven manipulation. The moves were badly needed, particularly at the EPA, after political interference during prior administrations derailed many determinations of dangers posed by toxic chemicals. A probe by the U.S. Government Accountability Office (GAO) found that the George W. Bush administration was involved in delaying EPA efforts to assess the public health risks of several chemicals, forcing EPA scientists to give drafts of scientific assessments to the White House's Office of Management and Budget (OMB) for review before they could be finalized. It was a requirement that ensured many such assessments never were completed. In fact, the OMB worked actively to kill several chemical assessments, the watchdog agency's investigation found. Making matters worse, the OMB's reviews of the EPA's scientific findings were dubbed secret, not to be shared with those most impacted—the public.

The GAO found undue political pressure was contaminating an EPA program called IRIS (Integrated Risk Information System), which catalogues scientific assessments and helps the EPA determine safe levels of chemical exposures. IRIS is "an important source of information on health effects that may result from exposure to chemicals in the environment," the GAO wrote in its report.[7] Investigators determined that though EPA scientists completed 32 draft assessments for chemical risks from 2006 to 2007, because of political interference only 4 were actually able to move forward and be finalized in the IRIS system. At the time of its report, in 2008, the GAO found that the 540 assessments that were completed in IRIS were rapidly becoming outdated, even as the EPA needed to be analyzing hundreds of other chemicals.

The EPA's IRIS assessment of how much glyphosate is safe for people to consume in food and water on a daily basis, for instance, was last revised in January 1987. The work was based on data provided by Monsanto.[8]

The revelations contained within the GAO's audit echoed the complaints of consumer and environmental advocates who had spent years watching the political pressure build and begging for someone to stop it. The Union of Concerned Scientists (UCS) summed up the situation this way:

EPA scientists apply their expertise to protect the public from air and water pollution, clean up hazardous waste, and study emerging threats such as global warming. Because each year brings new and potentially toxic chemicals into our homes and workplaces, because air pollution still threatens our public health, and because environmental challenges are becoming more complex and global, a strong and capable EPA is more important than ever. Yet challenges from industry lobbyists and some political leaders to the agency's decisions have too often led to the suppression and distortion of the scientific findings underlying those decisions—to the detriment of both science and the health of our nation.[9]

The UCS, a nonprofit founded in 1969 by scientists and students at the Massachusetts Institute of Technology, had more than the GAO audit to support its concerns. One month after the GAO issued its report, in March 2008, the UCS unveiled a devastating indictment of just how far the integrity of government scientists had fallen. The non-profit surveyed 3,400 scientists at the EPA, the FDA, and several other agencies about their levels of independence. The group found 1,301 scientists who said they feared retaliation if they expressed concerns about "mission driven work"; 688 scientists who reported they were unable to publish their work in peer-reviewed journals if it didn't adhere to agency policies; and 889 EPA scientists who had personally experienced "inappropriate interference" in their work. Nearly 400 scientists said they had witnessed EPA officials misrepresenting scientific findings; 284 said they had seen the "selective or incomplete use of data to justify a specific regulatory outcome"; and 224 scientists said they had been directed to "inappropriately exclude or alter technical information" in an EPA document. Nearly 200 of the respondents said they had been in situations in which they or their colleagues actively objected to or resigned from projects "because of pressure to change scientific findings." The UCS concluded: "Political appointees . . . have edited scientific documents, manipulated scientific assessments, and generally sought to undermine the science behind dozens of EPA regulations."[10]

The findings of the UCS survey were not much of a surprise. In 2004, David Lewis, a former senior-level research microbiologist with the EPA's Office of Research and Development, had gone before a congressional committee of the U.S. House of Representatives to blow the whistle on what he saw as corruption of the EPA's internal scientific research review process. Lewis, who spent thirty-one years at the EPA before resigning in 2003, said he had knowledge of situations in which the agency showed a "lack of integrity" that "clearly threatens public health and the environment." He said agency management passed off unreliable scientific data and erroneous conclusions in order to support certain political agendas. "EPA obviously has not achieved a reasonable separation between politics and objective science and fostered an open scientific debate," he told members of Congress.[11]

All of that was supposed to change under President Obama. And, for a while, people such as Washington, DC, attorney Jeff Ruch actually thought it might. Ruch had experienced firsthand what it felt like to be blackballed for trying to do what he thought was right as a government lawyer for the California legislature. It was one week before he was to be married, in December 1986, and part of his job at the time was to write an assessment of a state prison building project. Ruch had all sorts of concerns, primarily because the facility was to be located on ground so contaminated it would ultimately warrant the Superfund designation, reserved for the worst of our country's hazardous waste sites. His bosses wanted no mention of such concerns in his assessment, but he refused to omit them. He was fired. "I saw the fragility of professional ethics in public service," he recalled. "I also saw many people I thought were friends shrink away from me for fear of being tarred with my brush."

Ruch went on to work at the Government Accountability Project, a nonprofit whistle-blower protection group that exposed him to many people who had also experienced the political pressures that can come to bear on government scientists and other employees as they try to do their jobs. That insight led Ruch to cofound a nonprofit group called Public Employees for Environmental Responsibility, or PEER, in 1997 to champion the legal rights and integrity of those public employees. One of the group's top priorities is to combat the manipulation of science at public agencies and shield scientists whose research may run counter to moneymaking corporate interests. "An agency like EPA is constantly saying they're fine, their scientific integrity is above reproach," Ruch told me. "But the truth is, these agencies don't like inconvenient facts."[12]

Ruch was heartened to see Obama's office call for the establishment of scientific integrity policies at the regulatory agencies. The EPA's fourteen-page scientific integrity document enacted during the Obama administration sounded sincere. It called on scientific studies to be communicated to the public, the media, and Congress, "uncompromised by political or other interference." EPA managers were expressly prohibited from intimidating or coercing scientists to alter scientific data, findings, or their professional opinions. Similar policies were put in place at the USDA and other agencies.

But setting policies and following them are clearly two different things, and by the time Obama's two terms came to a close, PEER was again dealing with a steady stream of calls from government scientists complaining of bureaucratic meddling and censorship. Glyphosate and genetically modified organisms (GMOs), along with the insecticides suspected of causing honeybee die-offs, were all on a list of so-called sensitive subjects that government scientists said they were told they needed to be wary of weighing in on. The integrity policies that were supposed to have been established to protect employees were toothless efforts to paper over problems, with no significant impact, Ruch found.

Less than a month after the International Agency for Research on Cancer (IARC) linked glyphosate to cancer, PEER filed a legal petition with the USDA demanding that the agency do more to protect its own scientists, who increasingly were raising questions about the safety of farm chemicals, including glyphosate. Several scientists had complained to PEER lawyers that their research was being restricted and they were being subjected to retaliation for attempting to talk publicly about work they were doing that conflicted with agribusiness interests. The scientists were too afraid for their jobs to speak out about their complaints at that time, but in the winter of 2015, one did come forward as a whistle-blower. That scientist, an entomologist and agroecologist named Jonathan Lundgren, who had worked for the agency for eleven years, said that USDA managers had blocked publication of his research, barred him from talking to the media, and disrupted operations at the laboratory he oversaw after he tried to point out safety problems with a lucrative class of insecticides known as neonicotinoids that are sold by Bayer, Syngenta, and other big agrochemical companies. Two research reports by Lundgren concluded that farmers received no yield benefit at all in using the high-priced neonicotinoid seed treatments the companies were selling. His research also showed that neonicotinoids exacerbated conditions threatening the disappearing monarch butterfly population, but a supervisor told him the manuscript was "sensitive" and required elevated levels of approval, Lundgren said.

After agonizing for at least two years about whether or not to go public with what had happened, Lundgren filed a lawsuit against the agency in late 2015, resigning his post and putting a name and a face to the bigger problem of an agency under political influence. It was a difficult move for Lundgren, who had been considered a top USDA scientist and was named by President Obama as the recipient of a Presidential Early Career Award for Scientists and Engineers in 2011.

"There is a lot of fear in government scientists," Lundgren reflected. "If they don't fall into line, their science is torn apart and their personal lives are discredited. In my case, everyone that I cared about was either directly or indirectly attacked by the chain of command. Rules are selectively enforced to make the rogue scientist out to be a miscreant. Threats of criminal accusations are levied. These scientists are made an example of."

After Lundgren left the USDA, he and his wife, Jenna, retreated to a patch of prairie land in rural South Dakota, where Lundgren now conducts his research unfettered by political pressures. A group of area farmers and beekeepers helped him turn an old pole barn into a research facility, and a former dairy parlor where cows once were milked became his office. He spends his time focused on finding solutions for sustainable food systems.

"Drawing attention to oneself by doing controversial research is a quick way to draw ire and retaliation from the chain of command," he said. "But the world is facing some serious challenges right now, and we need science in areas like pollution, climate change, and our broken food production system. More than ever."[13]

A different USDA scientist, a veteran of the agency who specializes in plant health, has yet to find the courage to come forward with his concerns about glyphosate and the agrochemical industry. His work seems only mildly controversial, and it dovetails with that of others who fear the chemical is having long-term harmful effects on soil health. But because it runs directly counter to the positions of Monsanto and other industry players, he doesn't think he can risk speaking what he sees as the truth. "We have some pretty good research, but the USDA doesn't want to look at it," he told me, asking me to keep his identity a secret to protect his job.

When it comes to glyphosate, Monsanto clearly has seen the EPA as more ally than independent authority. A 2013 statement by the EPA concluding "that glyphosate does not pose a cancer risk to humans" has long graced a Monsanto web page, for instance. (The statement, posted in the *Federal Register*, was made as the EPA agreed to Monsanto's request to permit more glyphosate use on food crops and was based on data submitted by Monsanto.)

And immediately following IARC's announcement that its scientists had found glyphosate to be a probable human carcinogen, the company's expectation of EPA support was clear. Monsanto's Dan Jenkins, the company's key liaison to the EPA, scrambled to talk with agency officials, including Rowland, asking if the EPA would "correct the record"[14] and e-mailing the agency five pages of information to use in answering questions from the media.[15] The document provided guidance on how to discount the various studies showing links to non-Hodgkin lymphoma (NHL) and the tumors found in mice, and glyphosate detections in blood and urine, and it was shared among EPA staffers. The EPA has also dragged its feet on complying with Freedom of Information Act (FOIA) requests, failing to release thousands of pages of documents dealing with Monsanto and glyphosate.

It makes sense for Monsanto to seek to sway the agency in any way it can. After all, the EPA's judgment affects regulation both in the United States and abroad, and it is relied on by many farmers and consumers as the voice of authority on whether or not caution is required in using the chemical or consuming its residues in food and water. Moreover, the agency's assurances about glyphosate's safety give Monsanto an ace card in arguing that the individuals who are suffering from NHL and suing the company are wrong to believe their cancers were caused by Roundup.

Exactly how hard Monsanto or its surrogates pressured the EPA over glyphosate is unclear. Monsanto argues there was no improper agenda to push the EPA to issue a positive cancer review for the chemical. But attorneys for the people suffering from NHL say that buried within millions of internal Monsanto documents obtained through discovery is damning evidence demonstrating that the company has enjoyed a tight hold on the EPA for years. Exposing corporate influence is a key part of the legal strategy for those suing Monsanto. But the issue has a much broader significance, of course, because everyone using or consuming the chemical should expect thorough and impartial evaluations by regulators.

Though the story may take years to fully unfold, the early court filings in the Roundup litigation are both intriguing and highly concerning. They point not just to a close relationship between Monsanto and the EPA's Jess Rowland but to a culture of regulatory corruption and collusion with the chemical industry. One particularly damning document that has turned up—sent anonymously to lawyers for the cancer victims—is a letter addressed to Rowland from a fellow EPA scientist dated March 4, 2013, that accuses Rowland of playing "political conniving games with the science" to favor pesticide manufacturers such as Monsanto. "It is essentially certain that glyphosate causes cancer," states the letter, which came to light as evidence in the Roundup litigation. "For once do the right thing and don't make decisions based on how it affects your bonus."

The letter to Rowland carries the sign-off of thirty-year career EPA scientist Marion Copley, who left the agency in 2012 and died from breast cancer in 2014 at the age of sixty-six. The letter accuses Rowland of having "intimidated staff" to change reports to benefit industry, and it says that the scientific evidence surrounding glyphosate clearly shows the chemical should be categorized as a "probable human carcinogen," the same classification that IARC would make two years later. "I have cancer and I don't want these serious issues . . . to go unaddressed before I go to my grave," the Copley letter states.[16]

Longtime EPA scientist Evaggelos Vallianatos, a gregarious Greek who grew up on a small farm among olive groves in his home country and still speaks with a heavy Greek accent, said Monsanto has a long history of improper influence inside the EPA. During his twenty-five-year EPA stint from 1979 to 2004, he spent most of his time in the agency's Office of Pesticide Programs, where he saw repeated examples of what he believed to be clearly corrupt practices. It wasn't just Monsanto; the agency was nearly completely beholden to corporate interests, he remembers. "It's the pesticide merchants and GMO companies . . . they are the real decision makers," he said. "They use their lobbyists to shape national policy by almost buying politicians. It's this corruption that subverts the EPA. I am not a prophet, but I can see a very dark future if we fail to ban glyphosate and all other neurotoxins and carcinogens in our food and natural world."[17]

Vallianatos now writes and speaks publicly about what he says is a transformation of the EPA from a public watchdog to a "polluter's protection agency," and he cites numerous specific examples backed by EPA documents to support his claims. He compiled many of his observations in a 2014 book called *Poison Spring: The Secret History of Pollution and the EPA.*

Vallianatos sees Monsanto's actions to defend glyphosate as similar to the story line that played out during his time at the EPA over dioxins, the toxic chemical contaminants that were formed in the production of Monsanto's Agent Orange herbicide and other pesticides used in the United States and abroad. The EPA now acknowledges that dioxins are highly toxic and can cause cancer, reproductive and developmental problems, and damage to the immune system and can interfere with hormones. But for many years the agency aligned with Monsanto's assurances of dioxin's safety and relied in part on company-sponsored studies that showed human exposure to dioxin did not translate to increased cancer risks. Just as Monsanto has been trying to do with glyphosate, the company was able to leverage the EPA's inaction on dioxins to defend itself against legal claims. Those studies were suspected to be fraudulent by EPA chemist Cate Jenkins, and her accusations triggered the EPA to launch a criminal investigation of Monsanto. But after two years, the investigation was quietly closed, with no action against Monsanto.

Monsanto ultimately was not able to dodge the dioxin issue, however, agreeing in 2012 to commit more than $90 million for cleanup of dioxin contamination in Nitro, West Virginia, and for medical monitoring of Nitro residents who had been exposed to the company's contaminants. "The fear with dioxins was unprecedented toxicity. The strategy with glyphosate is protecting unprecedented profits," said Vallianatos.

Certainly, the EPA's job of overseeing the use of pesticides is not an easy one. As of September 2010, more than 16,000 pesticides were registered for use in the United States. That job is made harder by the fact that the agency's workforce has been in steady decline over the past two decades, dropping from more than 18,000 employees in 1999 to roughly 15,300 in 2016.[18] But still, the agency's scrutiny of pesticides allowed on the market has been deeply flawed. An investigation by the Natural Resources Defense Council (NRDC) found that most of those 16,000 pesticides were approved under what is known as "conditional" registration, a streamlined process meant to apply only in rare circumstances. Conditional registration allows products to enter the marketplace even though some of the required data may not have been submitted or reviewed by regulators. Chemical companies are supposed to provide all the needed data within certain time frames, but a review by the GAO determined that the EPA database designed to track these conditional registrations was a failure.[19]

"The American public may think all pesticides receive rigorous health and safety testing before they hit the shelves for sale. But our investigation shows their trust is misplaced," said the NRDC's Jennifer Sass. "The EPA has casually approved more than 10,000 pesticides for use in consumer products and in agriculture. . . . They've done so without transparency or public comment, and, in some cases, without toxicity tests to determine safety guidelines for public use."[20]

Questionable behavior by top agency officials has been seen time and again, particularly the prioritizing of secrecy over public accountability. Not only does the agency routinely fail to meet legal requirements for complying with FOIA requests to disclose records of its internal business, but top officials have also created alter ego e-mail addresses for conducting agency business, a practice that public interest groups feared was keeping agency work with corporate players away from the prying eyes of the public.

Obama's top agency chief, Lisa Jackson, for instance, was caught using an e-mail account with the name Richard Windsor to correspond with other government officials. The Competitive Enterprise Institute, a conservative Washington think tank, sued the Obama administration in 2012 for access to those e-mails, and Jackson subsequently resigned. The EPA has maintained that there is nothing nefarious about the extra e-mail accounts and that administrators commonly use e-mail addresses separate from those known to the public so they can more easily conduct business. The EPA has said these e-mails are available through the FOIA, just as the official e-mails are. Still, an investigation by the Associated Press found that many government officials use these secret e-mail accounts in ways that complicate an agency's legal responsibilities to find and turn over e-mails in response to congressional or internal investigations, civil lawsuits, or public records requests.[21]

The EPA's handling of the new herbicide that Dow brought to market combining 2,4-D with glyphosate also raised eyebrows. An investigation by the *Chicago Tribune* found that the EPA intentionally downplayed the risks of the new herbicide and ignored a law that required an extra safety factor to protect children's health. The *Tribune*'s Patricia Callahan discovered that EPA and Dow scientists had changed important analyses and a key measurement of toxicity in a pivotal rat study in ways that tweaked risk calculations just enough to allow for a dramatic increase in the use of the weed killer. Because much of the extra herbicide would be used on food crops, the EPA's changes meant that children in the United States could start consuming levels of 2,4-D—in combination with glyphosate—that the World Health Organization, Russia, Australia, South Korea, Canada, Brazil, and China considered unsafe.[22]

It's no secret that money talks in Washington. And it's no secret that Dow, Monsanto, and many others spread a lot of it around. CropLife America, whose stated mission is to promote agricultural pesticides on behalf of its membership of chemical companies, also is a generous donor to the policy makers who influence agricultural and pesticide policies. When it's all added up, many millions of dollars are spent each year on lobbying by the agrochemical companies and their associations. CropLife alone spends more than $2 million per year on lobbying, for instance.[23] The group also shelled out more than $260,000 in political contributions in 2016. And, according to research by the Center for Responsive Politics, agribusiness interests spent more than $127 million on lobbying[24] and donated more than $26.3 million to political campaigns in 2016, including those of several congressmen who are members of the House agriculture appropriations subcommittee.[25]

The organization frequently cites protection of farmers' interests when lobbying, but it is clear where its loyalties lie; its board of directors is composed not of farming groups but of multinational chemical companies. And in its role as the lobbying arm for the farm pesticide industry, CropLife has immense power in Washington, wielding it to "advance policy that highlights the vital role of pesticides." The EPA's acquiescence to CropLife's demands to remove Peter Infante from the Scientific Advisory Panel it convened on glyphosate in December 2016 was but one of many examples of CropLife's power and its efforts to influence the EPA. Top CropLife officials have served on advisory committees for the EPA and provided guidance on such matters of regulatory law as the Food Quality Protection Act, which deals with health-based standards for pesticides used in foods. CropLife has argued that a variety of laws aimed at providing clean water and protecting endangered species are unduly burdensome, as are rules that aim to reduce pesticide drift. CropLife has been a key player in delaying EPA action to remove the dangerous insecticide chlorpyrifos from the market, shrugging off the research showing the risks to children's brain development, and it has been a tireless champion of glyphosate safety, despite the many studies that indicate otherwise.

The organization has battled against EPA efforts to use epidemiology studies to analyze the safety of certain chemicals, instead telling the EPA it should continue to rely on industry-funded toxicology research.

And it has pushed back on EPA efforts to heed scientists' warnings that formulated herbicides, such as Roundup, may be more toxic than are the active ingredients alone. That strong-arming came in the summer of 2016, when the EPA said it was developing a research plan with the National Institute of Environmental Health Sciences to evaluate the role of glyphosate in product formulations and the "differences in formulation toxicity." Considering the growing body of independent science showing that product formulations—like Roundup—could be more dangerous than previously known, more research would seem to be an obvious move for the EPA. But not to CropLife. In a sharply worded letter to the EPA, the association criticized the agency for raising the concern and said that any data needed should come from the companies registering and selling the products.[26] The EPA then quietly backed off the plan.

"They want no regulations at all so they can make as much money as possible," said environmental lawyer Charlie Tebbutt, who has spent thirty years battling with chemical companies and organizations such as CropLife. He sees the agrochemical industry's substantial power over regulators and lawmakers as "business as usual," despite the obvious harm to people and the environment. "The public needs to know what they're doing behind the scenes," he said.[27]

There are real concerns that corporate influence could become even more pronounced during Donald Trump's presidency. Many of Trump's picks to oversee federal regulatory agencies have a record of siding with corporations on matters of public policy. Trump's advisors have pushed for large budget and staff cuts at the EPA, and, notably, Trump's pick to run the EPA, former Oklahoma attorney general Scott Pruitt, has a long history of fighting environmental regulation. As Oklahoma's attorney general, Pruitt sued the EPA several times over regulations dealing with air quality and pollution. He has primarily championed the interests of the oil and gas companies, which make up one of

Oklahoma's most economically powerful industries. But many fear that his affinity for industry will extend to the chemical companies peddling pesticides.

Even before Pruitt's nomination was approved by Congress, during the first week of the Trump administration, EPA scientists found themselves effectively gagged—ordered not to talk with the public or the press about their research. The EPA's public social media websites and press releases were frozen, and the communications director for Trump's EPA transition team announced that scientific reports generated by EPA scientists would be reviewed by political appointees before being made public. The actions sparked such a strong public backlash that the administration retreated and said there would be no such mandate.

The obvious efforts to suppress science prompted environmental activists to scale a crane located near the White House on Trump's fifth day in office and unfurl a large golden banner that featured black lettering proclaiming the message "RESIST."

Fears were realized only a few weeks into the new administration when Trump unveiled a budget plan that would slash the EPA's budget by 31 percent and cut roughly 3,000 employees from the agency. And the depths of allegiance to corporate interests was underscored when new EPA chief Pruitt overturned the agency's proposed ban on chlorpyrifos, handing a hard-fought victory to Dow AgroSciences, the chief purveyor of the insecticide. The move stunned and outraged environmental and consumer advocates because it had taken them years to get the EPA to acknowledge the evidence of the harm chlorpyrifos has on children's brain development. But over at the USDA, the move was applauded as a boon for farmers and agribusiness.[28] Critics noted that Dow's parent company, Dow Chemical, had donated $1 million to Trump's inauguration, and shortly after the contribution Trump chose Dow Chemical's chief executive officer to lead the American Manufacturing Council.[29]

If chlorpyrifos gets a pass, it's unlikely that glyphosate or any other highly profitable pesticide will get serious scrutiny by the EPA anytime soon.

Such moves by government agencies are unsettling, and the future of scientific independence and integrity is an open question as I write this. Former FDA chief Robert Califf, a cardiologist who left the agency when Trump took the White House, and who himself had been criticized as being too close to the pharmaceutical industry, stressed the need for a clear separation between politics and the work that should be done on behalf of the public. "Political appointees . . . should not be interfering," he said. "Once that happens for the wrong reason, how do you ever stop politics from dominating this arena?"[30]

In the view of Dr. Paul Winchester, medical director of the neonatal intensive care unit at the Franciscan St. Francis Health network in Indianapolis, Indiana, the EPA and other regulators are endangering generations of children by allowing pesticides such as glyphosate to become so pervasive. Research that he and other medical professionals are pursuing clearly shows correlations between pesticides found commonly in food and rising levels of chronic disease and neurodevelopmental problems in children as they grow into adults. He's outraged at what he sees as the EPA's complicity with corporations such as Monsanto to cover up the dangers of the pesticides they peddle. "This is a huge issue. We are convinced there is more than ample science to raise serious concerns over rising herbicide use and exposure, yet not nearly enough is being done to either dismiss such concerns or study them in a meaningful way. People think global warming is the biggest threat, but it's not. This is."[31]

CHAPTER 12
Seeking Solutions

If, having endured much, we have at last asserted our "right to know,"
and if, knowing, we have concluded that we are being asked to take senseless
and frightening risks, then we should no longer accept the counsel of those
who tell us that we must fill our world with poisonous chemicals; we should
look about and see what other course is open to us.

—Rachel Carson, *Silent Spring*

For Stephen Ellis, who grows wheat, barley, corn, and soybeans on 4,200 acres along Chesapeake Bay in Virginia, questions about glyphosate's safety and effectiveness are part of a broad risk-versus-reward ratio that he and other farmers must calculate as they confront the constant challenges Mother Nature brings.

Ellis has used glyphosate for decades, and though he has studied the reports of the links to disease, he knows that other herbicides are clearly more dangerous. Like other farmers, he uses paraquat, for instance, despite knowing that a few drops accidentally ingested can kill quickly. The chemical corrodes the gastrointestinal tract and leads to kidney, liver, and respiratory failure within days. Comparatively, the possibility that glyphosate may cause cancer years down the road is a risk he considers worth taking. And Ellis is a businessman who believes that his farm income has benefited greatly from glyphosate—once Roundup Ready crops came along and he could spray glyphosate directly onto growing corn, he was able to put land that had become overrun with weeds back into viable production. He also counts as a reward the fact that glyphosate use made it possible for him to avoid tilling the ground, which helped control erosion and chemical runoff into the waters of the bay. Before glyphosate resistance became a problem, "life was good and easy," Ellis recalled. Now, resistance is such an issue that he, like other farmers, is having to use additional chemicals to fight the weeds, and he is wondering how long glyphosate will last. Still, the chemical was a "godsend" for many years, he told me.[1]

For a lawyer like Charlie Tebbutt, who studies the impacts of chemical use on the environment and fights to hold companies and regulators accountable for pesticide problems, the fact that farmers have been big fans of glyphosate and other pesticides despite their harmful ramifications is not surprising. The chemical companies are "like the drug cartel warlords that get their people addicted to their drugs," he says. "They then argue that farmers need their products once they've hooked them."[2] Arguments by companies, such as Monsanto, of altruistic goals to feed the world are almost laughable; money is the driver and always has been, as far as Tebbutt is concerned. The global market for pesticides is valued at roughly $65 billion per year and growing, with the countries that make up the Americas the largest buyers.[3]

There is no doubt that many millions of farmers around the world have found rich benefits in glyphosate and other common agrochemicals and have come to believe that those rewards are more than worth the risks. Even if glyphosate were to be banned, or sharply restricted, as many people around the world have demanded, substitutes are just as dangerous, if not more so. Whether they are coated on seeds or sprayed from the ground or the air, pesticides have become ubiquitous in agriculture. Many farmers know no other way.

Our dependence on chemically based agriculture is an unfortunate truth, but so is the fact that the modern agricultural practices so highly dependent on synthetic pesticides simply are not sustainable over the long term—not if we want to protect the health of our families and our environment. There is simply too much evidence that pesticides contribute to elevated rates of chronic diseases such as different cancers, diabetes, neurodegenerative disorders that include Parkinson's disease and Alzheimer's disease, and reproductive disorders. Farmers are at higher risk because of their direct and repeated exposure to pesticides such as glyphosate and the many other herbicides, fungicides, and insecticides. But everyone who eats the foods produced with these pesticides is also at risk. And though the chemical agribusiness industry has long contended that low-level exposures pose no risk to human health, numerous scientists and medical professionals no longer are willing to accept that false assurance.

"Along with the wide use of pesticides in the world, the concerns over their health impacts are rapidly growing. There is a huge body of evidence on the relation between exposure to pesticides and elevated rate of chronic diseases such as different types of cancers, diabetes, neurodegenerative disorders like Parkinson, Alzheimer, and amyotrophic lateral sclerosis (ALS), birth defects, and reproductive disorders," an international team of toxicology experts wrote in a 2013 scientific research paper. The scientists said there also was circumstantial evidence on the association of pesticide exposure with asthma and chronic obstructive pulmonary disease and autoimmune diseases such as systemic lupus erythematous and rheumatoid arthritis. The scientists said improved policies for pesticide use were needed.[4]

Children are especially susceptible to the adverse effects of pesticides, as demonstrated by epidemiologic evidence of associations between early life exposure to pesticides and pediatric cancers, decreased cognitive function, and behavioral problems. And pesticide-laden diets, the snacks and cereals laced with weed- and bug-killing chemicals that so many of our children consume, are a big concern. More than seven years ago, in May 2010, scientists from the University of Montreal and Harvard University released a study showing that exposure to residues of pesticides commonly found on vegetables and fruit can double a child's risk of attention deficit hyperactivity disorder (ADHD), a condition that leaves kids with problems concentrating, hyperactivity, and impulse control issues.[5]

The 60,000-member American Academy of Pediatrics has been calling on regulators to strengthen pesticide oversight and take steps to better protect children, including the advancement of less toxic pesticide alternatives. The doctors' group is but one of numerous organizations representing medical professionals, scientists, consumers, environmentalists, and others who are demanding a healthier path forward.

So how do we get there? There are no easy answers, though many experts have ideas about how to start. Even some of the biggest agrochemical companies are beginning to acknowledge that new measures are needed for the future.

One partial solution may be found within the soil itself. In areas not ravaged by overuse of pesticides, a handful of soil can hold millions of microbes that carry rich traits to help plants grow better. Different traits interact with plants in different ways, but scientists have started harnessing and reproducing these beneficial microbes with the aim of converting them into commercial crop tools—sprays, coatings on seeds, and more—that could help crops resist disease and pests, absorb nutrients more efficiently, and generally improve overall plant health, quality, and yield. Industry leaders say they are working on treatments for corn and beans, wheat, canola, cotton, and many types of fruits and vegetables.

Some such "biologicals" have already been brought to market, with mixed but promising results. Many of the early generation of products combine microbials with synthetic pesticides, but the hope of many developers is that eventually the biologicals, which include both bio-pesticides and biostimulants, can stand on their own and that these more natural crop treatments can supplant harmful synthetic chemical offerings such as glyphosate. Because these microbial solutions are drawn from naturally occurring bacteria and fungi, they face far fewer consumer concerns and an accelerated path through the regulatory approval process.

Even the titans of the pesticide industry have jumped into the race to develop these new crop treatments, in recognition, no doubt, of the perilous future the current pesticide treadmill portends. The work started with small research and development firms, but as the potential value emerged, the big agricultural players quickly jumped in, buying up or partnering with the smaller firms. Monsanto tried to outpace competitors by testing more than 2,000 microbial strains at the same time on hundreds of thousands of field plots around the United States, a strategy Monsanto claims gives it the largest microbial research program in the world. The company partnered with a smaller biotech company called Novozymes in its quest to dominate the biologicals market, which analysts project at around $2 billion with a growth rate of 10–15 percent in the next few years. And though the company is careful not to criticize its own history of pushing harmful pesticides into the market, Monsanto's top scientist, Robb Fraley, calls the move badly needed.

"By working with a plant's own naturally-occurring processes, we have the potential to create products that are very precise and specific in how they work and may require smaller and fewer applications than current agricultural products," he said. "That's better for farmers, more sustainable and consistent with our vision to create products that enable farmers to produce more and conserve more."[6]

Jim Jones, assistant administrator for the EPA's Office of Chemical Safety and Pollution Prevention under President Barack Obama, has long been a big fan of the movement toward more biologically based crop applications. Jones spent twenty-six years as an EPA staffer working on chemical safety issues before being named by Obama to oversee the chemical safety office in 2013, so he has deep insider knowledge of the agency's strengths and weaknesses when it comes to protecting the public from pesticides. During a meeting in his office in the hulking EPA headquarters, he told me that the agency wanted to encourage the development of biopesticides because they "have very favorable human health and environmental profiles," and he predicted that they were likely to overtake synthetic chemicals in agriculture at some point. The EPA set up an approval system that was pushing the new biopesticides through in less than a year, compared with the two to three years or more it takes for many synthetic pesticides. The EPA also has offered reduced fees associated with registering biopesticides. "We're pretty bullish about them," Jones said. "We go out of our way . . . to express our enthusiasm for biopesticides."[7] Jones left the EPA with the transition to Donald Trump's team, but the biopesticide program continues.

The EPA defines biopesticides as products derived from natural materials such as animals, plants, bacteria, and certain minerals. The agency believes they are inherently less toxic than conventional pesticides and are safer for the people applying them. They also typically are effective in very small quantities and decompose quickly, reducing exposure and pollution problems. Biopesticides generally affect only the targeted pest and closely related organisms, in contrast to broad spectrum, conventional pesticides that may affect nontarget organisms such as birds, insects, and mammals.[8]

One example of how biopesticides can help farmers is seen in a naturally occurring single-cell yeast found on golden delicious apples and in the tissues of other plants. Scientists determined that this yeast could be isolated and applied to apples and pears after harvest to control particular fungal pathogens. Researchers have also developed products that rely on types of bacteria that attach to and infect or otherwise suppress types of roundworms that can be very damaging to strawberries and other fruit, vegetable, and field crops. In addition, scientists are discovering ways to arm plants to defend themselves against disease-carrying pathogens.

Overall, as I write this, the EPA has approved more than 430 biological active ingredients for use in pesticides. Use of these solely for U.S. agriculture is well over 4 million pounds now, compared with 900,000 pounds in 2000.

But while biologically based crop treatments may sound like a fast fix, there are several complications. To begin with, microbes that do their jobs well in certain soils and under certain climatic conditions don't necessarily function as hoped for when used in different settings. Living microbes often also need interaction with other specific organisms to function as desired, a dynamic that can complicate transitioning of the microbes into useful products. As well, concerns about toxicity don't completely disappear with microbial products, meaning thorough testing is still needed.

Matthew Wallenstein has been studying the complicated interplay of these invisible biological communities for years as a research scientist in the natural resource ecology laboratory at Colorado State University. Wallenstein, who holds a doctorate in ecology, is focusing his work on organisms that can enhance plant growth by improving nutrient uptake and enhancing soil health. He and two other Colorado State soil microbiologists started a company called Growcentia that sells organic soil supplements to enhance plant growth.

"We have an opportunity to continue to improve the productivity and efficiency of crop production by taking advantage of what nature has invented," he said. "Within a handful of soil you have a whole tropical rain forest worth of biodiversity, tens of thousands of different species that have evolved an incredible array of traits, and there is a huge potential to tap some of those natural abilities." But, he said, while "there is a lot of science in the lab that shows great potential, there are many remaining challenges to get it to work on millions of acres."[9]

What truly is needed to reduce pesticides and all the harm they create is a paradigm shift in the way we view food production and incentivize farmers. Rather than making a frenzied push for the cheapest and easiest crops to grow in a production system dependent on an arsenal of chemicals, we must set new priorities that emphasize long-term gains over short-term profits.

Some agricultural and policy experts say diverse organic agriculture is the model to pursue because it reduces pesticide use while creating nutritious food in a healthy environment. But converting a conventional farm to a certified organic operation can take years and exact a financial toll on farmers during the transition. The standards are fairly rigorous—organic farmers must demonstrate that they are protecting natural resources, conserving biodiversity, and using only approved substances on their farms. Consumer demand for organic foods has been rising steadily as consumers become more aware of the dangers of pesticides, pushing U.S. organic food sales to a record high of $43 billion in 2016.[10] Organic products are now available in nearly 20,000 natural food stores in the United States and nearly three out of four conventional grocery stores, with sales of organic products amounting to more than 5 percent of total U.S. food sales, according to recent industry statistics. Certified organic acreage and livestock have been expanding in the United States for many years, particularly for fruits, vegetables, dairy, and poultry, according to the U.S. Department of Agriculture (USDA).

Still, many consumers balk at paying the higher prices that typically are attached to organic products. And while there is a lot of research indicating that organic yields may come close to conventional ones, they often fall short of matching production levels achieved with pesticides, making it hard to convince conventional farmers to cast aside their long-relied-upon weed killers, insecticides, fertilizers, and fungicides. Organic industry advocates say they need more federal, state, and local programs to help support organic research. From 2002 to 2014, the USDA supplied roughly $142 million in research grants to address many components of organic agriculture, such as how to manage weeds adequately to sustain crop yields while protecting and building soil health.[11] But the investments will need to expand to bring organic production in line with consumer demand, organic industry leaders say.

An increasing number of environmental and agricultural experts say there is a middle ground—even if producers are not willing to take all the steps required to be considered an organic producer, they still can make changes that lower pesticide exposures and better protect people and the environment. Techniques that reduce the need for pesticides include planting cover crops, rotating different types of crops from season to season, using animal waste to fertilize fields, and creating large buffer zones around fields that offer diverse native plants. The buffer zones attract natural predators, such as birds, that will eat insects harmful to crops, which means farmers can cut down on insecticides. All the strategies help protect and replenish the soil, which is critical to long-term production of nutritious and abundant food supplies. "The hallmark of a truly sustainable system is its ability to regenerate itself. When it comes to farming, the key to sustainable agriculture is healthy soil, since this is the foundation for present and future growth," states a report by the Rodale Institute, which encourages and teaches sustainable farming practices.[12]

The term "agroecology" has come to define this effort to turn farming away from the resource-intensive, fossil-fueled, and pesticide-dependent practices tied to mass production of a few select crops, and instead toward a view of agricultural land as precious ecosystems to be pro-tected. Change will mean many things, including more research into agroecological techniques—such as strategies for fighting crop pests and diseases without pesticides—and into the breeding of enhanced varie-ties of important crops. Change also requires educating farmers about truly sustainable practices, which will be critical for the future of food production as the global population expands. The United Nations Food and Agriculture Organization is among many groups and individu-als around the world pushing agroecology initiatives as part of a badly needed turning point in the global food system.

To support such efforts, governments must shift subsidies and research funding from agro-industrial monoculture practitioners to small farm-ers using agroecological methods. There is no time to wait, according to Hilal Elver, who was appointed in 2014 as the United Nations' "special rapporteur," or designated independent expert, tasked with examining food and human rights issues across the globe. As a lawyer, research professor, and codirector of the Project on Global Climate Change, Human Security, and Democracy at the University of California, Santa Barbara, Elver has been among a number of international voices calling for systemic changes in agriculture. Industrialized agriculture is not only failing to feed the world but also contaminating the environment and poisoning its inhabitants, she and many others assert. "Agroecology is a traditional way of using farming methods that are less resource ori-ented, and which work in harmony with society," Elver said in a speech delivered in Amsterdam in 2014. "New research in agroecology allows us to explore more effectively how we can use traditional knowledge to protect people and their environment at the same time."[13]

Changing long-standing habits is hard. Some economists who study agricultural sustainability say that moving farmers from a focus on short-term production to long-term conservation would require finan-cial incentives from the government. These types of "green payments" to farmers who plant crops that are beneficial to the ecosystem have already started in the United States as a way to promote cover crops. The USDA's Natural Resources Conservation Service (NRCS) has been deploying teams of farmer/teachers across the country to convince farmers of the benefits of cover crops and to help spread the word that using them could earn a check from the government worth $40 to $60 per acre for up to three years. Farmers are told that adding crops such as oats, hay, rye, or buckwheat instead of using a steady rotation of corn and soybeans can enrich the soil substantially. The programs are making some progress but still lack robust government support. NRCS staffers are discouraged, for example, from touting the pesticide-reduction benefits that cover crops bring, and telling farmers to cut back on pesticides is frowned upon.

Without an overhaul of the current multibillion-dollar government system of farm subsidies, real change will be hard to come by. Since the 1930s, the United States has offered financial support to farmers to help them manage variations in weather, market prices, and other factors all aimed at ensuring a stable food supply, and such aid to U.S. farmers now amounts to billions of dollars each year through various programs. But support has historically been focused on only a few crops, including corn, soybeans, wheat, cotton, and rice, and usually has been skewed toward helping the largest and most financially secure farm operations, leaving more than half the nation's farmers without any type of farm subsidy. Thanks in part to those subsidies, we have an oversupply of many of these core crops. Take corn, for instance. U.S. government reports show that close to, or well over, a billion bushels of corn are left over from what gets used in America or sold overseas each year.[14] Corn growers, not coincidentally, typically use a variety of high-priced pesticides in their operations that translate to hefty profits for agrochemical companies. There clearly is ample room for a shift in priorities and funding.

Greg Stegner, a lifelong Missouri farmer and a resource conservationist with the USDA's NRCS, has made a series of changes on his own 500-acre farm that show the benefits of cover cropping and cutting back on pesticides. He tries to convince other farmers that while more work may be involved in some of the practices, the long-term payoffs are worthwhile. Younger farmers want to listen, while the older ones tend to want to stick with what they know works, he said. Government incentives are confusing and often contradictory, Stegner said, and remain too focused on prioritizing farmers to focus on growing crops such as corn. "I've realized our government programs aren't really here to help us farmers much," he said. "It's about cheap food for the population . . . and profits for the big corporations."[15]

Perhaps most critically, we need immediate, widespread reform of our regulatory system. Transparency at all levels is vital. Corporate influence over regulators must be curtailed, and safety data on pesticide products can no longer be secreted away from the scrutiny of the public and of independent scientists. A responsible government cannot rely on safety testing that is conducted by self-interested corporations but must support research performed by truly independent academic and government scientists. This work could be funded by a registration tax on each new pesticide that a company wants to bring to market. And when it comes to determining what, if any, safe levels exist for pesticide residues in food, regulators should depend not on corporate-generated science, as they currently do, but on robust independent research that takes into account cumulative exposures people face each day in this pesticide-laden world.

The FDA and the USDA should accept the recommendations of the U.S. Government Accountability Office (GAO) and start routinely testing food products for glyphosate residues as long as the weed killer remains widely used on food crops. It is unconscionable that the primary agencies consumers must rely on for food safety guidance have spent decades declining to test for possible contamination of such a pervasive crop chemical. The lack of action is especially egregious considering that the agencies have known for years about research linking glyphosate to cancer and other diseases. At the very least, U.S. regulators need to let the public know what other common pesticides are used on food but not tested for each year, along with the potential effects of not testing. The GAO recommended as much to the agencies in 2014, but the advice was ignored.[16]

The EPA must also start robust evaluations of formulated products rather than focusing safety assessments on single active ingredients. Instead of looking solely at glyphosate, for instance, regulators must give greater consideration to what people are actually exposed to—finished products such as Roundup. And much more research is needed on the cumulative impacts of the range of pesticides people are exposed to regularly. The fact that a single strawberry sample contains residues of more than a dozen different pesticides cannot be brushed aside as inconsequential.

It is time for the EPA to make good on its obligation to identify and restrict endocrine-disrupting pesticides to protect people as well as fish and wildlife. The Food Quality Protection Act requires that the EPA screen pesticide chemicals for their potential as endocrine disruptors, extremely damaging hormone-altering chemicals that can cause cancerous tumors, birth defects, and other developmental disorders. But despite the 1996 legal requirement for the EPA to identify and act, the agency has accomplished little in the past two decades plus. The EPA's Office of Inspector General castigated the agency in 2011 for lack of action, but the agency continues to drag its feet on identifying and restricting these dangerous types of pesticides.

The precautionary principle should be the guide. It is not always realistic or safe to wait until science is completely settled. When there is evidence of harm, when corporate proclamations conflict with independent experts' views, the protection of people and the planet must take priority. There is no doubt that the pervasive pesticides in our lives come with risks and rewards, and balancing the interests of industry and individuals is a delicate endeavor. But too often regulators have shown a willingness to err on the side of business rather than on the side of caution. That must change.

This new path will require a cultural shift in the way we view farming and food production, and it could very likely translate to higher food prices, at least in the near term as conventional farmers shift their practices. But extra pennies for pesticide-free, or at least pesticide-reduced, foods is a small price to pay for healthier food, a healthier environment, reductions in illness and disease, and a brighter future for our children.

The damage already accrued to the environment and to individual lives cannot be undone. But the evidence of the dangers of glyphosate and other agrochemicals can no longer be suppressed, can no longer be whitewashed. The time to act is now. Some steps forward are small; others require a more aggressive stride. But we cannot stand still.

"Innovation does not happen without the courage to question the current paradigm," said Jonathan Lundgren, the former USDA scientist who left the agency when he felt his scientific findings were being sacrificed for political purposes. "If we do not change our behavior, then humans are in trouble. We know what needs to be done to solve these problems that our planet and species are facing. What is lacking is the courage to implement the needed changes."[17]

Let's find the courage.

Epilogue

Teri McCall doesn't like to talk much about her lawsuit against Monsanto. Even as the litigation slogs forward, as lawyers thumb through millions of documents, studies, memos, and reports, and as expert witnesses prepare their testimonies for the long-winding case that may take years to resolve, McCall is trying to move past her pain. Doing so has been made harder by the fact that she was diagnosed with early-stage breast cancer shortly after losing Jack. She tackled the cancer with aggressive surgery and now considers that fight also part of her past. Still, she has lost weight; the slim blue jeans and soft blouses she favors hang loose on her limbs. Her blue eyes and honey-blond hair still have the brightness of a woman decades younger, but her face has gained shadows of grief that she is not sure will ever be erased.

She remains haunted by the final months of Jack's failed struggle to survive. After a tumor on his neck was removed, the wound refused to heal and became infected. The chemotherapy and radiation treatments left him with burns and with a loss of taste, taking away even the enjoyment of his life's work, the fruits of the orchard outside his bedroom window.

"I felt like we were the healthiest of people," McCall said. She had never before worried about her food much, but now she does, fearing glyphosate or other types of pesticide residues. And she had never known how fast devastation could descend. "It's just overwhelming when you are going through this," she told me. "It's a horror story, to get cancer."

After Jack's death, she decided she would buy a horse, learn to ride, anything that was new, that might offer a fresh diversion from memories of her life with Jack. She measured out land next to the house for a corral and started daydreaming of the escape that conquering a new skill might bring. Her own cancer diagnosis and treatment, coming even as she still faced stacks of Jack's medical bills, added painful complications to an already excruciating effort to build a new life.

To help make ends meet, Teri rented out a garage apartment to a longtime girlfriend and reopened her home to traveling strangers as an occasional bed-and-breakfast. She encourages her guests to relax on the wide front porch, where she and Jack used to sit at the end of long days to talk and stare at the stars.

"He loved life, he loved people. He would want me to be happy," she said, leaning back on a floral sofa in the farmhouse front room that is positioned to catch afternoon sunlight. Next to her, a rectangular white pillow is stitched with the words "Love You Forever."

"I am trying. I am. I know I had a really good life, and I am thankful I had him for forty years," she says. "We used to hold hands in bed every night. Who has that?"[1]

At Jack's funeral, his son Paul delivered what he called an "artistic eulogy" memorializing his father's life and his early death. It was a piercingly personal tribute, but this much can be shared:

A cosmic monarch flew south across a desert valley garden, and when had reached the sea perched upon a man reading the red letters of Luke, a man whose heart wished to speak. A man thinking of every man. A man whose shell was starting to melt.

He had answers to a child's question. . . . With the faith of a child and dimpled serenity, a mind spinning in infinity, he had answers.

He rode waves. . . . The agrarian waves of Santa Rosa creek he rode, cultivating foremost faith, then love, then apples, children . . . joy. He rode a perfect point break in Baja, naked and on a full moon. He rode a pure and unhindered love for a certain woman.

He lives on. He lives on. He lives on in that friend some of us have that dares and dreams and speaks their wild mind of love without fear of judgment. He lives on in the creamy comfort of an avocado. He lives on in the post office, friendly exchanges and anywhere love is practiced. He lives on in the mystic church of many central coast hearts and hearts abroad. His spirit lives on in heaven, his thumbprint lives on in the community and his voice and image live on in the dreams of a son.

A cosmic monarch flew south across a desert garden and when had reached the sea perched upon a man reaching the red letters of Luke. The man shed his earthly shell, was transfigured and began to float away. And being guided by the monarch ascended into the heavens. And having had a desire to share his heart with us a phrase was written in the sand. "Love each other."[2]

Acknowledgments

Much love and gratitude go to my endlessly patient husband, Don, who gave me the "Go Away, I'm Writing!" sign that hangs in my office and who provided limitless support and encouragement over the many long months of writing. And to my amazingly unselfish children, Ally, Andrew, and Ryan, who allowed me the space and peace to bring the words to the pages, and who I fervently hope will find a better, cleaner, healthier future. Many thanks also to the brilliance of Gary Ruskin and Stacy Malkin, the fearless duo who founded U.S. Right to Know and forged the path that led to many of the revelations in these pages. I also owe more than I can say to the editors, colleagues, extended family members, and friends who helped keep me on track, pushed me to do more, to dig deeper, and to "stick to the facts." Here is but a partial list: Peter Bohan; Kim Bradford; Toni Cardarella; Nick Carey; Dan Margolies; Julia Sobek; Emily Turner; my father, Chuck Gillam; and my much-loved mother, Carol Heiss, who tirelessly read and reread each chapter. None of this work could have been accomplished without the many farmers and scientists (far too many to mention by name) who have taught me so much over the years and helped guide my inquiries into the story behind the spin. And finally, I am so grateful to the countless individuals—mothers, fathers, teachers, doctors, and others—who have reached out to tell me their stories and to ask me to find answers to their questions. Thank you all.

Notes

Introduction: A Silent Stalker

1. Joseph F. Rinella, Pixie A. Hamilton, and Stuart W. McKenzie, "Persistence of the DDT Pesticide in the Yakima River Basin, Washington," U.S. Geological Survey Circular 1090, p. 9, https://pubs.usgs.gov/circ/1993/1090/report .pdf.

2. Stephen B. Powles, "Gene Amplification Delivers Glyphosate-Resistant Weed Evolution," *Proceedings of the National Academy of Sciences of the United States of America* 107, no. 3 (January 19, 2010): 955–956, doi:10.1073 /pnas.0913433107.

3. Charles M. Benbrook, "Trends in Glyphosate Herbicide Use in the United States and Globally," *Environmental Sciences Europe* 28, no. 3 (February 2, 2016), doi:10.1186/s12302-016-0070-0.

4. Douglas Main, "Glyphosate Now the Most-Used Agricultural Chemical Ever," *Newsweek*, February 2, 2016, http://www.newsweek.com/glyphosate -now-most-used-agricultural-chemical-ever-422419.

Chapter 1: What Killed Jack McCall?

1. Comments and quotes in this chapter by Teri McCall and Paul McCall are from a discussion with the author on March 23, 2016.

2. J. Ferlay et al., GLOBOCAN 2012 v1.0, Cancer Incidence and Mortality Worldwide: IARC Cancer Base No. 11 (Internet) (Lyon, France: International Agency for Research on Cancer), 2013, http://www.wcrf.org/int /cancer-facts-figures/worldwide-data; American Cancer Society, "What Are the Key Statistics about Non-Hodgkin Lymphoma?," https://www.cancer

.org/cancer/non-hodgkin-lymphoma/about/key-statistics.html, last revised January 6, 2017.

3. World Health Organization, International Agency for Research on Cancer, *Evaluation of Five Organophosphate Insecticides and Herbicides*, IARC Monographs vol. 112, March 20, 2015, http://www.iarc.fr/en/media-centre/iarcnews/pdf/MonographVolume112.pdf.

4. Lin Fritschi, in conversation with the author, October 2016.

5. Teri Michelle McCall v. Monsanto Company, Case No. 3:16-cv-05749-VC in the U.S. District Court for the Central District of California, March 9, 2016, https://usrtk.org/wp-content/uploads/2017/02/Teri-McCall-lawsuit.pdf.

6. The Estate of Robert Cochran by Misty Hill, Its Administrator v. Monsanto Company, Case No. 3:17-cv-00293 DRH-SCW in the U.S. District Court for the Southern District of Illinois, filed March 20, 2017, p. 35, https://jnswire.s3.amazonaws.com/jns-media/47/f8/535559/RobertCochran.pdf.

7. Carey Gillam, "Monsanto Weed Killer Deserves Deeper Scrutiny as Scientific Manipulation Revealed," *Huffington Post*, March 17, 2017, http://www.huffingtonpost.com/entry/monsanto-weed-killer-deserves-deeper-scrutiny-as-scientific_us_58cc5541e4b0e0d348b34348.

8. Thomas F. Armstrong (Monsanto), memorandum to Robert J. Taylor (EPA), February 9, 1987, https://archive.epa.gov/pesticides/chemicalsearch/chemical/foia/web/pdf/103601/103601-230.pdf.

9. Robert D. Coberly (EPA), memorandum to Lee TerBush (EPA), February 11, 1974, https://archive.epa.gov/pesticides/chemicalsearch/chemical/foia/web/pdf/103601/103601-009.pdf.

10. Christine Sheppard, in conversation with the author, October 2016.

11. Enrique Rubio v. Monsanto Company, Case No. 2:15-cv-07246-DMG-E in the U.S. District Court for the Central District of California, Western Division, filed September 22, 2015, p. 6.

12. Carey Gillam, "Monsanto Says Panel to Review WHO Finding on Cancer Link to Herbicide," Reuters, July 14, 2015, http://www.reuters.com/article/us-monsanto-herbicide-idUSKCN0PO2FM20150714.

13. William Dykstra and George Z. Ghali (EPA), memorandum to Robert Taylor and Lois Rossi (EPA), October 30, 1991, p. 1, https://archive.epa.gov

/pesticides/chemicalsearch/chemical/foia/web/pdf/103601/417300-1991
-10-30a.pdf.

14. Attorney General of the State of New York, Consumer Frauds and Protection Bureau, Environmental Protection Bureau, "In the Matter of Monsanto Company, Respondent, Assurance of Discontinuance Pursuant to
Executive Law § 63(15), New York, NY, November 1996: False Advertising by Monsanto Regarding the Safety of Roundup Herbicide (Glyphosate)," p. 4, http://big.assets.huffingtonpost.com/fraud.pdf.

15. Aaron Johnson, in conversation with the author, November 2016.

16. Associated Press, "$700 Million Settlement in Alabama PCB Lawsuit,"
New York Times, August 21, 2003, http://www.nytimes.com/2003/08/21
/business/700-million-settlement-in-alabama-pcb-lawsuit.html.

17. Patrick McCreless, "New Anniston Study Shows Possible Link between
PCBs and Liver Disease," *Anniston (AL) Star*, October 21, 2016, http://www
.annistonstar.com/news/anniston/new-anniston-study-shows-possible
-link-between-pcbs-and-liver/article_2a625476-97d3-11e6-a7c0-c78
d019a1f2b.html.

18. Don Huber, in conversation with the author, August 2016.

19. Environmental Working Group, "National Drinking Water Database:
Glyphosate Exposure by State," http://www.ewg.org/tap-water/chemical
-contaminants/Glyphosate/2034/.

20. Statement issued by Harrington Investments in response to a query from
the author, August 19, 2016.

Chapter 2: An Award-Winning Discovery

1. Gerald M. Dill et al., "Glyphosate: Discovery, Development, Applications,
and Properties," in *Glyphosate Resistance in Crops and Weeds: History, Development, and Management*, ed. Vijay K. Nandula (Hoboken, NJ: John
Wiley & Sons, 2010), p. 1.

2. Ernst Schönbrunn et al., "Interaction of the Herbicide Glyphosate with
Its Target Enzyme 5-Enolpyruvylshikimate 3-Phosphate Synthase in Atomic
Detail," *Proceedings of the National Academy of Sciences of the United States
of America* 98, no. 4 (February 13, 2001): 1376–1380, doi:10.1073/pnas
.98.4.1376.

3. U.S. Patent Office, "3,799,758, N-Phosphonomethyl-Glycine Phytotoxicant Compositions, John E. Franz, Crestwood, Mo., assignor to Monsanto Company, St. Louis, Mo."

4. National Science & Technology Medals Foundation, "John E. Franz: National Medal of Technology and Innovation, Agriculture, 1987," http://www.nationalmedals.org/laureates/john-e-franz.

5. Stephen B. Powles, "Gene Amplification Delivers Glyphosate-Resistant Weed Evolution," *Proceedings of the National Academy of Sciences of the United States of America* 107, no. 3 (January 19, 2010): 955–956, doi:10.1073/pnas.0913433107.

6. Monsanto Company, "Biography of Dr. John Franz," https://web.archive.org/web/20080724175539/http://www.monsanto.com/features/franz_bio.asp.

7. Nick Visser, "Monsanto Advocate Says Roundup Is Safe Enough to Drink, Then Refuses to Drink It," *Huffington Post*, March 27, 2015, http://www.huffingtonpost.com/2015/03/27/monsanto-roundup-patrick-moore_n_6956034.html.

8. Monsanto Company, "Glyphosate Isn't a Beverage; Patrick Moore Isn't a Monsanto Lobbyist," *Beyond the Rows* (blog), March 27, 2015, http://monsantoblog.com/2015/03/27/glyphosate-isnt-a-beverage-patrick-moore-isnt-a-monsanto-lobbyist/.

9. U.S. Geological Survey, U.S. Bureau of Land Management, and U.S. Department of Agriculture, Forest Service, *Development of Phosphate Resources in Southeastern Idaho: Draft Environmental Impact Statement* (Reston, VA: U.S. Geological Survey, U.S. Bureau of Land Management, and U.S. Department of Agriculture, Forest Service, 1976), p. 1-8.

10. Stephen O. Duke and Stephen B. Powles, "Glyphosate: A Once-in-a-Century Herbicide," *Pest Management Science* 64, no. 4 (online version dated February 13, 2008): 319–325, doi:10.1002/ps.1518, https://www.researchgate.net/publication/228666854_Mini-review_Glyphosate_a_once-in-a-century_herbicide.

11. Dennis C. Williams, "The Guardian: EPA's Formative Years, 1970–1973," September 1993, EPA Web Archive EPA-202-K-93-002, https://archive.epa.gov/epa/aboutepa/guardian-epas-formative-years-1970-1973.html.

12. William Sanjour, in conversation with the author, July 15, 2016.

13. U.S. Environmental Protection Agency, "R.E.D. Facts: Glyphosate," EPA Reregistration Eligibility Decision EPA-738-F-93-011, September 1993, p. 4, https://archive.epa.gov/pesticides/reregistration/web/pdf/0178 fact.pdf.

14. Ibid., p. 2.

15. U.S. Environmental Protection Agency, Office of Pesticides and Toxic Substances, memorandum titled "Consensus Review of Glyphosate, Caswell No. 661A," March 4, 1985, https://www3.epa.gov/pesticides/chem _search/cleared_reviews/csr_PC-103601_4-Mar-85_171.pdf.

16. Ibid.

17. William Dykstra (EPA), memorandum to Hoyt Jamerson (EPA), February 10, 1984, https://archive.epa.gov/pesticides/chemicalsearch/chemical/foia /web/pdf/103601/103601-166.pdf.

18. U.S. Environmental Protection Agency, "Risk Assessment for Carcinogenic Effects," https://www.epa.gov/fera/risk-assessment-carcinogens.

19. George J. Levinskas (Monsanto), memorandum to T. F. Evans, April 3, 1985, https://usrtk.org/wp-content/uploads/2017/05/MDL1985mouseslide memo.pdf.

20. Nancy Beiles, "What Monsanto Knew," *The Nation*, May 11, 2000, https:// www.thenation.com/article/what-monsanto-knew/.

21. Robert Sauer, "Pathology Working Group Report on Glyphosate in CD-1 Mice," Pathco Inc., October 10, 1985.

22. Stephen L. Johnson (FIFRA Scientific Advisory Panel), memorandum to Steven Schatzow (EPA), February 24, 1986, https://archive.epa.gov/pesticides /chemicalsearch/chemical/foia/web/pdf/103601/103601-209.pdf.

23. William Dykstra (EPA), memorandum to Robert J. Taylor (EPA), June 19, 1989, https://usrtk.org/wp-content/uploads/2017/05/EPA-on-mouse-study -repoeatHQ_0000612.pdf.

24. Dennis P. Ward (Monsanto), letter to Robert J. Taylor (EPA), December 12, 1988, https://usrtk.org/wp-content/uploads/2017/05/EPA-on-mouse-study -repoeatHQ_0000612.pdf.

25. William Dykstra and George Z. Ghali (EPA), memorandum to Robert Taylor and Lois Rossi (EPA), October 30, 1991, p. 1, https://www3.epa.gov /pesticides/chem_search/cleared_reviews/csr_PC-103601_30-Oct-91 _265.pdf.

26. "3-Ex Officials of Major Laboratory Convicted of Falsifying Drug Tests," *New York Times*, October 22, 1983, http://www.nytimes.com/1983/10/22 /us/3-ex-officials-of-major-laboratory-convicted-of-falsifying-drug-tests. html.

27. Ellen Griffith Spears, *Baptized in PCBs: Race, Pollution, and Justice in an All-American Town* (Chapel Hill: University of North Carolina Press, 2014), pp. 156–157.

28. Cate Jenkins (EPA), memorandum to John West and Kevin Guarino (EPA), November 15, 1990, http://www.pbs.org/pov/stories/vietnam/discuss/38 /post.5.

29. E. G. Vallianatos and McKay Jenkins, *Poison Spring: The Secret History of Pollution and the EPA* (New York: Bloomsbury Press, 2014), pp. 63–66.

30. Douglas Foster and Mark Dowie, "The Illusion of Safety—Part One: Poisoned Research," *Mother Jones*, June 1982, p. 45.

31. U.S. Environmental Protection Agency, Office of Prevention, Pesticides and Toxic Substances, "Reregistration Eligibility Decision (RED): Glyphosate," September 1993, Appendix C, pp. C-3–C-37, http://static1.square space.com/static/5338c313e4b0cb384b4b7995/t/56526443e4b0a376ef8 50828/1448240195891/1993+epa+glyphosate+RED.pdf.

32. Nathan Donley, scientist with the Center for Biological Diversity, in conversation with the author, July 20, 2016.

33. U.S. Environmental Protection Agency, Office of Pesticides and Toxic Substances, Office of Pesticide Programs, "Environmental Fact Sheet: Risk/ Benefit Balancing under the Federal Insecticide, Fungicide, and Rodenticide Act," February 1990, https://nepis.epa.gov/Exe/ZyPURL.cgi?Dockey =9100CFR2.TXT.

34. U.S. Environmental Protection Agency, Office of Prevention, Pesticides and Toxic Substances, "Reregistration Eligibility Decision (RED): Glyphosate," September 1993, Appendix C, pp. C-3–C-37, http://static1.square space.com/static/5338c313e4b0cb384b4b7995/t/56526443e4b0a376ef8 50828/1448240195891/1993+epa+glyphosate+RED.pdf.

35. Maxie Jo Nelson (EPA), memorandum to R. Taylor and V. Walters (EPA), March 22, 1989, https://archive.epa.gov/pesticides/chemicalsearch /chemical/foia/web/pdf/103601/103601-245.pdf.

36. U.S. Environmental Protection Agency, "R.E.D. Facts: Glyphosate," EPA-738-F-93-011, September 1993, p. 4, https://www3.epa.gov/pesticides /chem_search/reg_actions/reregistration/fs_PC-417300_1-Sep-93.pdf.

37. Arthur Grube et al., U.S. Environmental Protection Agency, Office of Chemical Safety and Pollution Prevention, Office of Pesticide Programs, Biological and Economic Analysis Division, "Pesticides Industry Sales and Usage: 2006–2007 Market Estimates," February 2011, p. 12, https://www .epa.gov/sites/production/files/2015-10/documents/market_estimates 2007.pdf.

Chapter 3: The "Roundup Ready" Rollout

1. Monsanto Company, "Petition for Determination of Nonregulated Status: Soybeans with a Roundup Ready Gene," September 14, 1993, p. 29, https://www.aphis.usda.gov/brs/aphisdocs/93_25801p.pdf.
2. Mark Nelson, in conversation with the author, July 26, 2016.
3. Monsanto Company, "Petition for Determination of Nonregulated Status: Soybeans with a Roundup Ready Gene," September 14, 1993, p. 2, https://www.aphis.usda.gov/brs/aphisdocs/93_25801p.pdf.
4. Ibid.
5. Ibid.
6. Monsanto Company, "Selected Financial Data," fiscal year 2000, p. 24, http://www.monsanto.com/investors/pages/sec_html.aspx?xid=1361529 &vid=aHR0cDovL2FwaS50ZW5rd2l6YXJkLmNvbS9maWxpbmcue G1sP2lwYWdlPTEzNjE1MjkmRFNFUT0xMiZTRVE9JlNRREVTQ z1TRUNUSU9OX0VYSElCSVQmZXhwPSZzdWJzaWQ9NTc=&com pId=122069.
7. Monsanto Company, "2001 Annual Report," p. 32, http://www.annual reports.com/HostedData/AnnualReportArchive/m/NYSE_MON_2001 .pdf.
8. Texas Grain Storage, Inc. v. Monsanto Company, Case No. 5:07-cv-00673 -OLG-PMA in the U.S. District Court for the Western District of Texas, filed August 10, 2007.
9. Christopher Leonard, "Monsanto Uses Patent Law to Control Most of U.S. Corn, Soy Seed Market," Associated Press, December 16, 2009, http://www .cleveland.com/nation/index.ssf/2009/12/monsanto_uses_patent_law _to_co.html.
10. U.S. Government Accountability Office, "Genetically Engineered Crops: Agencies Are Proposing Changes to Improve Oversight, but Could Take Additional Steps to Enhance Coordination and Monitoring; Highlights,"

GAO-09-60, November 5, 2008, http://www.gao.gov/products/GAO-09-60.

11. Supreme Court of the United States, Monsanto Co. et al. v. Geertson Seed Farms et al., decided June 21, 2010, https://www.supremecourt.gov/opinions/09pdf/09-475.pdf.

12. Supreme Court of the United States, dissent by Justice J. Stevens in Monsanto Co. et al. v. Geertson Seed Farms et al., p. 20, https://www.supremecourt.gov/opinions/09pdf/09-475.pdf.

13. Center for Food Safety, et al. v. Thomas J. Vilsack and Monsanto Company, et al., Case No. 10-17719 in the U.S. Court of Appeals for the Ninth Circuit, http://cases.justia.com/federal/appellate-courts/ca9/10-17719/10-17719-2011-03-10.pdf?ts=1411052867.

14. Ruling in Center for Food Safety, et al. v. Thomas Vilsack, et al., Case No. C-08-00484 JSW in the U.S. District Court for the Northern District of California, https://drive.google.com/file/d/0B-pJR4cGo9ckTDlSVU1nMDJ0dTg/view?usp=sharing.

15. Tadlock Cowan and Kristina Alexander, "Deregulating Genetically Engineered Alfalfa and Sugar Beets: Legal and Administrative Responses," Congressional Research Service, September 10, 2012, https://www.agri-pulse.com/ext/resources/pdfs/c/r/s/e/t/CRS-GE-Alfalfa-Sugarbeet.pdf.

16. Erika Engelhaupt, "Government Pesticide and Fertilizer Data Dropped," *Environmental Science & Technology* 42, no. 18 (2008): 6779–6780, doi:10.1021/es801937k.

17. Charles Benbrook, in conversation with the author, August 8, 2016.

18. Jef Smidts (Andre & CIE, Antwerp), memorandum titled "Reflections about Bio-Engineered Wheat Possibly Introduced by Monsanto."

19. U.S. Environmental Protection Agency, memorandum titled "Updated Screening Level Usage Analysis (SLUA) Report for Glyphosate," October 22, 2015, https://drive.google.com/file/d/0B-pJR4cGo9ckb3k4UDczbVdiT1E/view.

20. Ibid.

Chapter 4: Weed Killer for Breakfast

1. Home-Grown Cereals Authority (HGCA), "Pre-harvest Glyphosate Application to Wheat and Barley," Information Sheet 02, Summer 2008,

http://cereals.ahdb.org.uk/media/185527/is02-pre-harvest-glyphosate
-application-to-wheat-and-barley.pdf.

2. Jason Vanfossan (USDA), e-mail to Terry Councell (FDA), August 29, 2014,
https://usrtk.org/wp-content/uploads/2017/05/GIPSA-wheawt.png.

3. Alliance for Natural Health USA, "Glyphosate Levels in Breakfast Foods:
What Is Safe?," April 19, 2016, http://www.anh-usa.org/wp-content/up
loads/2016/04/ANHUSA-glyphosate-breakfast-study-FINAL.pdf.

4. GMO Free USA, "GMO Free USA Finds GMOs and Weedkiller in Kellogg's Froot Loops," press release, January 29, 2015, http://www.csrwire.com
/press_releases/37644-GMO-Free-USA-Finds-GMOs-and-Weedkiller-in
-Kellogg-s-Froot-Loops.

5. Fernando Rubio, Emily Guo, and Lisa Kamp, "Survey of Glyphosate Residues in Honey, Corn and Soy Products," *Journal of Environmental & Analytical Toxicology* 5 (November 19, 2014): 249, doi:10.4172/2161-0525
.1000249.

6. Bruce Hemming, in conversation with the author, April 2015.

7. U.S. Geological Survey, Environmental Health–Toxic Substances Hydrol-
ogy Program, "Common Weed Killer Is Widespread in the Environment,"
April 23, 2014, http://toxics.usgs.gov/highlights/2014-04-23-glyphosate
_2014.html.

8. William Battaglin, in conversation with the author, August 2016.

9. William A. Battaglin et al., "Glyphosate and Its Degradation Product
AMPA Occur Frequently and Widely in U.S. Soils, Surface Water, Groundwater, and Precipitation," *Journal of the American Water Resources Association* 50, no. 2 (2014): 275–290, doi:10.1111/jawr.12159.

10. Michael Hansen, in conversation with the author, August 2016.

11. U.S. Environmental Protection Agency, "Glyphosate—Pesticide Petition
(PP#2E7979)," Docket ID: EPA-HQ-OPP-2012-0132, https://www.regu
lations.gov/docket?D=EPA-HQ-OPP-2012-0132.

12. Environmental Protection Agency, "Final Rule, Glyphosate; Pesticide Tolerances," *Federal Register* 78, no. 84 (May 1, 2013): 25396–25401, https://
www.gpo.gov/fdsys/pkg/FR-2013-05-01/pdf/2013-10316.pdf.

13. Ibid.

14. Ibid.

15. Gary M. Williams, Robert Kroes, and Ian C. Munro, "Safety Evaluation
and Risk Assessment of the Herbicide Roundup and Its Active Ingredi-

ent, Glyphosate, for Humans," *Regulatory Toxicology and Pharmacology* 31, no. 2 (April 2000): 117–165, doi:10.1006/rtph.1999.1371.

16. Marie Sønnegaard Poulsen et al., "Modeling Placental Transport: Correlation of *In Vitro* BeWo Cell Permeability and *Ex Vivo* Human Placental Perfusion," *Toxicology in Vitro* 23, no. 7 (October 2009): 1380–1386, doi: 10.1016/j.tiv.2009.07.028.

17. David Murphy and Henry Rowlands, "Glyphosate: Unsafe on Any Plate," Food Democracy Now! and the Detox Project, November 14, 2016, https://s3.amazonaws.com/media.fooddemocracynow.org/images/FDN _Glyphosate_FoodTesting_Report_p2016.pdf.

18. Moms Across America, "EPA Admits Widespread Misuse of Roundup Herbicide Must Stop," press release, April 19, 2016, http://www.momsacross america.com/press_release.

19. Organic Consumers Association, Moms Across America, and Beyond Pesticides v. General Mills Inc., Case No. 2016 CA 006309 B in the Superior Court of the District of Columbia, http://www.beyondpesticides.org /assets/media/documents/2016.08.24NatureValleyDCCourtStamped Complaint.pdf.

20. U.S. Department of Agriculture, Agricultural Marketing Service, Science and Technology Program, "Pesticide Data Program: Annual Summary, Calendar Year 2014," https://www.ams.usda.gov/sites/default/files/media /2014%20PDP%20Annual%20Summary.pdf.

21. U.S. Department of Agriculture, Agricultural Marketing Service, Pesticide Data Program, "PDP Special Projects," https://www.ams.usda.gov/datasets /pdp/pdp-special-projects.

22. U.S. Department of Agriculture, Agricultural Marketing Service, Science and Technology Program, "Pesticide Data Program: Annual Summary, Calendar Year 2011," p. 25 and Appendix C, https://www.ams.usda.gov/sites /default/files/media/2011%20PDP%20Annual%20Summary.pdf.

23. Diana Haynes (USDA), e-mail to staffers titled "April–June 2017 PDP Program Plan," January 11, 2017.

24. Carey Gillam, "USDA Drops Plan to Test for Monsanto Weed Killer in Food," *Huffington Post*, March 23, 2017, http://www.huffingtonpost.com /entry/usda-drops-plan-to-test-for-monsanto-weed-killer-in_us_58d2d b4ee4b062043ad4af84.

25. Kimberly Hodge-Bell, "Concerned about Pesticide Residue?," Monsanto Company, *Beyond the Rows* (blog), April 1, 2015, http://monsantoblog.com /2015/04/01/concerned-about-pesticide-residue/.

26. R. W. Cook (EPA), memorandum to R. J. Taylor and Toxicology Branch (EPA) titled "Glyphosate on Wheat Grain and Straw: Evaluation of Analytical Methods and Residue Data," January 22, 1991, https://archive.epa .gov/pesticides/chemicalsearch/chemical/foia/web/pdf/103601/103601 -260.pdf.

27. U.S. Food and Drug Administration, "Total Diet Study," http://www.fda .gov/Food/FoodScienceResearch/TotalDietStudy/default.htm.

28. Timothy H. Begley (FDA), e-mail to Michael E. Kashtock (FDA) titled "Methods for Pesticide Coverage," January 17, 2013, http://usrtk.org/wp -content/uploads/2016/09/FDA3.pdf.

29. U.S. Government Accountability Office, "Food Safety: FDA and USDA Should Strengthen Pesticide Residue Monitoring Programs and Further Disclose Monitoring Limitations," GAO-15-38, October 2014, http://www .gao.gov/assets/670/666408.pdf.

30. Laura Bowman, in conversation with the author, July 2016.

31. Canadian Food Inspection Agency, "Safeguarding with Science: Glyphosate Testing in 2015–2016," April 2017, https://usrtk.org/wp-content /uploads/2017/04/CFIA_ACIA-9123346-v1-FSSD-FSSS-Glyphosate -Final-Report-15-16_018410-1.pdf.

32. U.S. Department of Agriculture, "Pesticide Data Program: Annual Summary, Calendar Year 2015," https://www.ams.usda.gov/sites/default/files /media/2015PDPAnnualSummary.pdf.

33. Ibid., p. 16.

34. Chensheng Lu, in conversation with the author, November 2016.

35. Alice Park, "Exposure to Pesticides in Pregnancy Can Lower Children's IQ," *Time*, April 21, 2011, http://healthland.time.com/2011/04/21/exposure-to -pesticides-in-pregnancy-can-lower-childrens-iq/.

36. Virginia A. Rauh et al., "Brain Anomalies in Children Exposed Prenatally to a Common Organophosphate Pesticide," *Proceedings of the National Academy of Sciences of the United States of America* 109, no. 20 (April 20, 2012): 7871–7876, doi:10.1073/pnas.1203396109.

37. European Parliamentary Research Service, "Human Health Implications of Organic Food and Organic Agriculture," Science and Technology Options

Assessment PE 581.922, December 2016, http://www.europarl.europa.eu
/RegData/etudes/STUD/2016/581922/EPRS_STU(2016)581922_EN
.pdf.

38. Ibid., p. 6.

39. Harvard T.H. Chan School of Public Health, Q&A with Philippe
Grandjean, February 8, 2017, https://www.hsph.harvard.edu/news/features
/health-benefits-organic-food-farming-report/.

40. International Food Information Council Foundation, "Food Decision
2016: Food and Health Survey," http://www.foodinsight.org/sites/default
/files/2016-Food-and-Health-Survey-Report_FINAL1.pdf.

41. Danielle S. Cooper v. The Quaker Oats Company, Case No. 3:16-cv
-02364 in the U.S. District Court for the Northern District of California,
https://assets.documentcloud.org/documents/2820643/Quaker-Oats
-Class-Action-Complaint.pdf.

42. Lee I-chia, "FDA Says Pesticide Residue Found in 10 Oatmeal Items," *Tai-
pei Times*, May 27, 2016, http://www.taipeitimes.com/News/front/archives
/2016/05/27/2003647215.

43. Monsanto Company, "Preharvest Staging Guide," p. 3, https://usrtk.org/wp
-content/uploads/2016/09/Monsanto-application-guide-for-preharvest
.pdf.

44. Ibid., p. 10.

45. Carey Gillam, "FDA to Start Testing for Glyphosate in Food," *Time*,
February 17, 2016, http://time.com/4227500/fda-glyphosate-testing/?xid
=fbshare.

46. Internal e-mails and reports obtained through Freedom of Information Act
request FDA #2016-717.

47. Ibid.

48. Nate Carmichael, in conversation with the author, September 2016.

49. Marcela Carmichael, in conversation with the author, September 2016.

50. Margaret Lombard, in conversation with the author, September 2016.

51. Amelia Jackson-Gheissari (Monsanto), e-mail to Lauren Robin (FDA),
April 15, 2016, http://usrtk.org/wp-content/uploads/2016/09/FDA4.pdf.

52. Narong Chamkasem (FDA) and Gary Hinshaw (USDA), e-mail exchange,
May 5, 2015.

53. Jay Feldman, in conversation with the author, September 2016.

54. Michael Antoniou, in conversation with the author, September 2016.

Chapter 5: Under the Microscope

1. Vera Lúcia de Liz Oliveira Cavalli et al., "Roundup Disrupts Male Reproductive Functions by Triggering Calcium-Mediated Cell Death in Rat Testis and Sertoli Cells," *Free Radical Biology and Medicine* 65 (December 2013): 335–346, doi:10.1016/j.freeradbiomed.2013.06.043.

2. Robin Mesnage et al., "Multiomics Reveal Non-alcoholic Fatty Liver Disease in Rats Following Chronic Exposure to an Ultra-Low Dose of Roundup Herbicide," *Scientific Reports* 7 (January 2017): 39328, doi:10.1038/srep39328.

3. Jessica Nardi et al., "Prepubertal Subchronic Exposure to Soy Milk and Glyphosate Leads to Endocrine Disruption," *Food and Chemical Toxicology* 100 (February 2017): 247–252, doi:10.1016/j.fct.2016.12.030.

4. Alejandra Paganelli et al., "Glyphosate-Based Herbicides Produce Teratogenic Effects on Vertebrates by Impairing Retinoic Acid Signaling," *Chemical Research in Toxicology* 23, no. 10 (August 9, 2010): 1586–1595, doi:10.1021/tx1001749.

5. Michael Warren and Natacha Pisarenko, "Birth Defects, Cancer in Argentina Linked to Agrochemicals: AP Investigation," Associated Press, October 21, 2013, http://www.ctvnews.ca/health/birth-defects-cancer-in-argentina-linked-to-agrochemicals-ap-investigation-1.1505096.

6. Channa Jayasumana et al., "Drinking Well Water and Occupational Exposure to Herbicides Is Associated with Chronic Kidney Disease, in Padavi-Sripura, Sri Lanka," *Environmental Health* 14, no. 6 (January 18, 2015), doi:10.1186/1476-069X-14-6.

7. Nihal Jayatilake et al., "Chronic Kidney Disease of Uncertain Aetiology: Prevalence and Causative Factors in a Developing Country," *BMC Nephrology* 14, no. 180 (August 2013), doi:10.1186/1471-2369-14-180.

8. U.S. Patent Office, "No. 3,160,632: Aminomethylenephosphinic Acids, Salts Thereof, and Process for Their Production," Stauffer Chemical Company, December 8, 1964.

9. Channa Jayasumana, Sarath Gunatilake, and Priyantha Senanayake, "Glyphosate, Hard Water, and Nephrotoxic Metals: Are They the Culprits Behind the Epidemic of Chronic Kidney Disease of Unknown Etiology in Sri Lanka?," *International Journal of Environmental Research and Public Health* 11, no. 2 (2014): 2125–2147, doi:10.3390/ijerph110202125.

10. Kristin Wartman Lawless, "No One Knows Exactly How Much Herbicide Is in Your Breakfast," *VICE* Media, May 11, 2016, http://www.vice.com/read /no-one-knows-how-much-herbicide-is-in-your-breakfast.

11. Siriporn Thongprakaisang et al., "Glyphosate Induces Human Breast Cancer Cells Growth via Estrogen Receptors," *Food and Chemical Toxicology* 59 (September 2013): 129–136, doi:10.1016/j.fct.2013.05.057.

12. Céline Gasnier et al., "Glyphosate-Based Herbicides Are Toxic and Endocrine Disruptors in Human Cell Lines," *Toxicology* 262, no. 3 (August 21, 2009): 184–191, doi:10.1016/j.tox.2009.06.006.

13. Nicolas Defarge et al., "Co-formulants in Glyphosate-Based Herbicides Disrupt Aromatase Activity in Human Cells below Toxic Levels," *International Journal of Environmental Research and Public Health* 13, no. 3 (February 26, 2016): 264, doi:10.3390/ijerph13030264.

14. Nora Benachour and Gilles-Eric Séralini, "Glyphosate Formulations Induce Apoptosis and Necrosis in Human Umbilical, Embryonic, and Placental Cells," *Chemical Research in Toxicology* 22, no. 1 (2009): 97–105, doi: 10.1021/tx800218n.

15. World Health Organization, International Agency for Research on Cancer, *Evaluation of Five Organophosphate Insecticides and Herbicides*, IARC Monographs vol. 112, March 20, 2015, p. 79, http://monographs.iarc.fr /ENG/Monographs/vol112/mono112-09.pdf.

16. Pesticide Action Network International, "The Glyphosate Monograph," October 2016, p. 4, http://issuu.com/pan-uk/docs/glyphosate_monograph _complete?e=28041656/43997864.

17. Paul Winchester, MD, report to 2017 Children's Environmental Health Translational Research Conference, Arlington, VA, April 5, 2017.

18. Leah Schinasi and Maria E. Leon, "Non-Hodgkin Lymphoma and Occupational Exposure to Agricultural Pesticide Chemical Groups and Active Ingredients: A Systematic Review and Meta-Analysis," *International Journal of Environmental Research and Public Health* 11, no. 4 (April 2014): 4449–4527, doi:10.3390/ijerph110404449.

19. National Cancer Institute, Surveillance, Epidemiology, and End Results Program, "Cancer Stat Facts: Non-Hodgkin Lymphoma," https://seer.cancer .gov/statfacts/html/nhl.html.

20. Michael C. R. Alavanja et al., "Non-Hodgkin Lymphoma Risk and Insecticide, Fungicide, and Fumigant Use in the Agricultural Health Study," *PLOS One*, October 22, 2014, doi:10.1371/journal.pone.0109332.

21. A. J. De Roos et al., "Integrative Assessment of Multiple Pesticides as Risk Factors for Non-Hodgkin's Lymphoma among Men," *Occupational and Environmental Medicine* 60, no. e11 (2003), doi:10.1136/oem.60.9.e11, http://www.occenvmed.com/cgi/content/full/60/9/e11.

22. Lennart Hardell and Mikael Eriksson, "A Case-Control Study of Non-Hodgkin Lymphoma and Exposure to Pesticides," *Cancer* 85, no. 6 (March 15, 1999): 1353–1360, doi:10.1002/(SICI)1097-0142(19990315)85:6<1 353::AID-CNCR19>3.0.CO;2-1.

23. Helen H. McDuffie et al., "Non-Hodgkin's Lymphoma and Specific Pesticide Exposures in Men: Cross-Canada Study of Pesticides and Health," *Cancer Epidemiology, Biomarkers & Prevention* 10, no. 11 (November 2001): 1155–1163, http://cebp.aacrjournals.org/content/10/11/1155.full-text.pdf.

24. John Peterson Myers et al., "Concerns over Use of Glyphosate-Based Herbicides and Risks Associated with Exposures: A Consensus Statement," *Environmental Health* 15, no. 19 (February 17, 2016), doi:10.1186/s12940 -016-0117-0.

25. Ibid.

26. Monsanto Company, "Monsanto Transitions away from Tallowamine in Products," blog posting, April 8, 2016, http://monsantoblog.eu/monsanto -transitions-away-from-tallowamine-in-products-enfr/#.

27. Monsanto Company, "Glyphosate Safety by the Numbers," http://news .monsanto.com/image/infographic/glyphosate-safety-numbers.

28. Gary M. Williams, Robert Kroes, and Ian C. Munro, "Safety Evaluation and Risk Assessment of the Herbicide Roundup and Its Active Ingredient, Glyphosate, for Humans," *Regulatory Toxicology and Pharmacology* 31, no. 2 (April 2000): 117–165, doi:10.1006/rtph.1999.1371.

29. William Heydens (Monsanto), e-mail to Donna Farmer (Monsanto), February 19, 2015, https://usrtk.org/wp-content/uploads/2017/03/Heydens.png.

30. U.S. District Court for the Northern District of California, In Re: Roundup Products Liability Litigation, Case No. 3:16-md-02741-VC, Document 226-3, Filed April 6, 2017, p. 2, https://usrtk.org/wp-content/uploads/2017 /04/226series.pdf.

31. Monsanto executives, e-mail thread, July 2012, https://tpin.webaction.org /c/79/images/Monsanto%20collusion%20with%20dow,%20syngenta .pdf.

32. Larry D. Kier and David J. Kirkland, "Review of Genotoxicity Studies of Glyphosate and Glyphosate-Based Formulations," *Critical Reviews in Toxicology* 43, no. 4 (2013): 283–315, doi:10.3109/10408444.2013.770820.

33. U.S. Public Interest Research Group, "Monsanto Colluded to 'Ghost-Write' Studies on the Pesticide Roundup," press release, March 15, 2017, http://www.uspirg.org/news/usp/monsanto-colluded-ghost-write-studies -pesticide-roundup.

34. Monsanto Company, "What Is Glyphosate?," http://www.monsanto.com /sitecollectiondocuments/glyphosate-safety-health.pdf.

35. Anneclaire J. De Roos et al., "Cancer Incidence among Glyphosate-Exposed Pesticide Applicators in the Agricultural Health Study," *Environmental Health Perspectives* 113, no. 1 (January 2005; published online November 4, 2004): 49–54, doi:10.1289/ehp.7340.

36. Aaron Blair, in conversation with the author, March 2015.

37. World Health Organization, International Agency for Research on Cancer, *IARC Monographs on the Evaluation of Carcinogenic Risks to Humans*, vol. 112, *Some Organophosphate Insecticides and Herbicides*, published online 2015, updated August 2016, pp. 77–79, http://monographs.iarc.fr/ENG /Monographs/vol112/mono112-10.pdf.

38. Francesco Forastiere, in conversation with the author, September 2016.

39. International Agency for Research on Cancer, "Preamble to the IARC Monographs," Section B (6), http://monographs.iarc.fr/ENG/Preamble/current b6evalrationale0706.php.

40. Christopher Portier, in conversation with the author, September 2016.

41. Donna Farmer, "What the IARC 2A Rating for Glyphosate Really Means," *Beyond the Rows* (Monsanto Company blog), March 20, 2015, http://mon santoblog.com/2015/03/20/what-the-iarc-2a-rating-for-glyphosate-really -means/.

42. Daniel Jenkins (Monsanto), e-mail to Michael Goodis (EPA), March 23, 2015.

43. Philip Miller (Monsanto), letter to Margaret Chen (WHO), March 20, 2015.

44. Christopher Wild (IARC), letter to Philip Miller (Monsanto), April 16, 2015.

45. Howard Minigh (CropLife International), letter to Margaret Chen (WHO) and Christopher Wild (IARC), May 13, 2015.

46. Monsanto Company internal report, "Proposal for Post-IARC Meeting Scientific Projects Draft," Case No. 3:16-md-02741-VC in the U.S. District Court for the Northern District of California, Document 187-5, May 11, 2015, p. 1.

47. Carey Gillam, "Monsanto Says Panel to Review WHO Finding on Cancer Link to Herbicide," Reuters, July 14, 2015, http://www.reuters.com/article/us-monsanto-herbicide-idUSKCN0PO2FM20150714.

48. Monsanto Company v. Office of Environmental Health Hazard Assessment and Lauren Zeise, Case No. 16-CECG-00183 in the Superior Court of the State of California, County of Fresno, http://www.monsanto.com/files/documents/monvoehha.pdf.

49. Francesco Forastiere, in conversation with the author, September 2016.

50. Sharon Lerner, "EPA Used Monsanto's Research to Give Roundup a Pass," *The Intercept*, November 3, 2015, https://theintercept.com/2015/11/03/epa-used-monsanto-funded-research/.

51. Jess Rowland (EPA), memorandum to Charles Smith and Khue Nguyen (EPA) titled "Glyphosate: Report of the Cancer Assessment Review Committee," October 1, 2015, http://www.acsh.org/wp-content/uploads/2016/05/EPA-glyphosate-document-final.pdf.

52. U.S. Environmental Protection Agency, Office of Research and Development, "Summary of ORD Comments on OPP's Glyphosate Cancer Assessment," December 14, 2015, https://usrtk.org/wp-content/uploads/2017/03/ORDcommentsonOPPglyphosate.pdf.

53. William Dykstra and Jess Rowland (EPA), memorandum to Melba Morrow (EPA), April 20, 1998, https://archive.epa.gov/pesticides/chemicalsearch/chemical/foia/web/pdf/103601/103601-1998-04-20a.pdf.

54. Daniel J. Jenkins (Monsanto), e-mail to William F. Heydens (Monsanto), April 28, 2015, https://usrtk.org/wp-content/uploads/2017/03/JessRowlandseries.pdf.

55. Jess Rowland (EPA), memorandum to Charles Smith and Khue Nguyen (EPA) titled "Glyphosate: Report of the Cancer Assessment Review

Committee," October 1, 2015, http://www.acsh.org/wp-content/uploads/2016/05/EPA-glyphosate-document-final.pdf.

56. Daniel J. Jenkins (Monsanto), e-mail to Tracey L. Reynolds (Monsanto), September 3, 2015, https://usrtk.org/wp-content/uploads/2017/03/JessRowlandseries.pdf.

57. Plaintiffs' Motion to Compel Deposition of Jess Rowland, Case No. 3:16-md-02741-VC in the U.S. District Court for the Northern District of California, Document 189, filed March 14, 2017, https://usrtk.org/wp-content/uploads/2017/03/JessRowlandseries.pdf.

58. Plaintiffs' Reply in Further Support of Motion to Compel Responses from Deponent Jesudoss Rowland, Case No. 3:16-md-02741-VC in the U.S. District Court for the Northern District of California, Document 284, filed May 10, 2017, https://usrtk.org/wp-content/uploads/2017/05/MDLPlaintiffsreplyonRowlanddepo.pdf.

59. U.S. Environmental Protection Agency, Office of Pesticide Programs, "Glyphosate Issue Paper: Evaluation of Carcinogenic Potential," September 12, 2016, https://www.epa.gov/sites/production/files/2016-09/documents/glyphosate_issue_paper_evaluation_of_carcincogenic_potential.pdf.

60. Monsanto Company, internal document titled "Glyphosate," Case No. 3:16-md-02741-VC in the U.S. District Court for the Northern District of California, Document 189-5, p. 2.

61. Monsanto Company, "The EPA's Registration Review of Glyphosate," http://www.monsanto.com/pages/epa-review-of-glyphosate.aspx.

62. Janet E. Collins (CropLife America), letter to Steven Knott (EPA), August 24, 2016, http://191hmt1pr08amfq62276etw2.wpengine.netdna-cdn.com/wp-content/uploads/2016/01/Final-CLA-Glyphosate-SAP-08-24-16.pdf.

63. Janet E. Collins (CropLife America), letter to Steven Knott (EPA), October 12, 2016, http://191hmt1pr08amfq62276etw2.wpengine.netdna-cdn.com/wp-content/uploads/2016/01/CLA-Comments-on-SAP-Disqualification-10-12-16.pdf.

64. Carey Gillam, "EPA Bows to Chemical Industry in Delay of Glyphosate Cancer Review," *Huffington Post*, October 19, 2016, http://www.huffingtonpost.com/carey-gillam/epa-bows-to-chemical-indu_b_12563438.html.

65. Peter Infante, in conversation with the author, October 2016.

66. Peter Infante, in conversation with the author, December 2016.

67. Steve Davies, "Glyphosate Panel Split on Chemical's Carcinogenicity," Agri-Pulse Communications, December 16, 2016, http://www.agri-pulse.com /Glyphosate-science-panel-split-on-chemicals-carcinogenicity-12162016 .asp#.WFWBBpLGV94.twitter.

68. Vicky Laybourne, in conversation with the author, January 2016.

69. U.S. Environmental Protection Agency, memorandum with SAP Final Report, March 16, 2017, https://www.epa.gov/sites/production/files/2017-03 /documents/december_13-16_2016_final_report_03162017.pdf.

70. Thierry Vrain, in conversation with the author, March 2016.

71. Ibid.

Chapter 6: Spinning the Science

1. Nathaniel Rich, "The Lawyer Who Became DuPont's Worst Nightmare," *New York Times*, January 6, 2016, https://www.nytimes.com/2016/01/10 /magazine/the-lawyer-who-became-duponts-worst-nightmare.html.

2. Eric S. Sachs (Monsanto), e-mail to a group of professors titled "Invitation to Author a Policy Brief in the Series 'Perspectives on Science Matters,'" August 8, 2013, pp. 31, 33, https://assets.documentcloud.org/documents /2303692/david-shaw-missstateuniverdocs.pdf.

3. Tom Philpott, "These Emails Show Monsanto Leaning on Professors to Fight the GMO PR War," *Mother Jones*, October 2, 2015, http://www.mother jones.com/tom-philpott/2015/09/monsanto-professors-gmo-PR.

4. Laura Krantz, "Harvard Professor Failed to Disclose Connection," *Boston Globe*, October 1, 2015, http://www.bostonglobe.com/metro/2015/10/01 /harvard-professor-failed-disclose-monsanto-connection-paper-touting -gmos/lLJipJQmI5WKS6RAgQbnrN/story.html.

5. Nora Benachour and Gilles-Eric Séralini, "Glyphosate Formulations Induce Apoptosis and Necrosis in Human Umbilical, Embryonic, and Placental Cells," *Chemical Research in Toxicology* 22, no. 1 (2009): 97–105, doi: 10.1021/tx800218n.

6. GMOSeralini, "What Were the Study's Findings?," http://www.gmoseralini .org/faq-items/what-were-the-studys-findings/.

7. Gilles-Eric Séralini et al., "Republished Study: Long-Term Toxicity of a Roundup Herbicide and a Roundup-Tolerant Genetically Modified Maize," *Environmental Sciences Europe* 26, no. 14 (June 24, 2014), doi:10.1186 /s12302-014-0014-5.

8. Susan Bardocz et al., "Seralini and Science: An Open Letter," *Independent Science News*, October 2, 2012, https://www.independentsciencenews.org/health/seralini-and-science-nk603-rat-study-roundup/.

9. Carey Gillam, "Keeping Secrets from Consumers: Labeling Law a Win for Industry-Academic Collaborations," *Huffington Post*, July 14, 2016, https://usrtk.org/uncategorized/keeping-secrets-from-consumers-labeling-law-a-win-for-industry-academic-collaborations/.

10. E-mail exchanges dated November 2012 obtained by U.S. Right to Know, https://www.usrtk.org/wp-content/uploads/2016/07/Goodman-Nov.-22012RG-000664-000001.pdf.

11. Carey Gillam, "Keeping Secrets from Consumers: Labeling Law a Win for Industry-Academic Collaborations," *Huffington Post*, July 14, 2016, https://usrtk.org/uncategorized/keeping-secrets-from-consumers-labeling-law-a-win-for-industry-academic-collaborations/; e-mail exchanges dated November 2012 obtained by U.S. Right to Know, https://www.usrtk.org/wp-content/uploads/2016/07/GoodmanRG-000126-000001.pdf.

12. GMOSeralini, "Editor of Food and Chemical Toxicology Is Obliged to Give Prof. Séralini's Team Right of Reply after Retracting NK603 and Roundup Study," May 19, 2014, http://www.gmoseralini.org/editor-of-food-and-chemical-toxicology-is-obliged-to-give-prof-seralinis-team-right-of-reply-after-retracting-nk603-and-roundup-study/.

13. Gilles-Eric Séralini, "Why Glyphosate Is Not the Issue with Roundup: A Short Overview of 30 Years of Our Research," *Journal of Biological Physics and Chemistry* 15, no. 3 (2015): 111–119, doi:10.4024/12SE15R.jbpc.15.03, http://www.gmoseralini.org/wp-content/uploads/2015/11/Seralini-career-JBPC_2015.pdf.

14. Channa Jayasumana et al., "Drinking Well Water and Occupational Exposure to Herbicides Is Associated with Chronic Kidney Disease, in Padavi-Sripura, Sri Lanka," *Environmental Health* 14, no. 6 (January 18, 2015), doi:10.1186/1476-069X-14-6.

15. Rick Goodman, Daniel Goldstein, and John Vicini, e-mail exchanges, October 6–7, 2014, catalogued by U.S. Right to Know, https://www.usrtk.org/wp-content/uploads/2016/07/GoodmanSriLanka1RG-000010-000001.pdf.

16. Carey Gillam, "The True Inside Story of How a College Professor Sells Out to Monsanto," AlterNet, January 30, 2016, http://www.alternet.org/food/true-inside-story-how-college-professor-sells-out-monsanto.

17. Internal Revenue Service Form 990 filings by Council for Biotechnology Information, 2014, 2015.
18. Henry Miller and Bruce Chassy, "Scientists Smell a Rat in Fraudulent Genetic Engineering Study," *Forbes*, September 25, 2012, http://www.forbes .com/sites/henrymiller/2012/09/25/scientists-smell-a-rat-in-fraudulent -genetic-engineering-study/#7f0c8c1c1ff1.
19. Eric Sachs and Bruce Chassy, e-mail exchanges, September 13, 2011, obtained by U.S. Right to Know, https://www.usrtk.org/wp-content/uploads /2016/01/BruceChassy4.pdf.
20. Eric Sachs and Bruce Chassy, e-mail exchanges, January 2012, catalogued by *Mother Jones*, https://www.motherjones.com/files/chassychina.pdf.
21. Bruce Hammond and Bruce Chassy, e-mail exchanges, April 24, 2012, obtained by U.S. Right to Know, https://www.usrtk.org/wp-content/uploads /2016/01/BruceChassy6.pdf.
22. Bruce Chassy, e-mail to Gregory Knott (University of Illinois), October 20, 2010, obtained by U.S. Right to Know, https://www.usrtk.org/wp-content /uploads/2016/01/BruceChassy10-1.pdf.
23. Bruce Chassy and Eric Sachs, e-mail exchange, October 19, 2011, obtained by U.S. Right to Know, https://www.usrtk.org/wp-content/uploads /2016/01/BruceChassy11.pdf.
24. Bruce Chassy and Sheryl Evertowski, e-mail exchange, October 19, 2011, obtained by U.S. Right to Know, https://www.documentcloud.org/documents /2303693-bruce-chassyuofillinoisdocs.html.
25. Monica Eng, "Why Didn't an Illinois Professor Have to Disclose GMO Funding?," WBEZ, March 15, 2016, https://www.wbez.org/shows/wbez -news/why-didnt-an-illinois-professor-have-to-disclose-gmo-funding /eb99bdd2-683d-4108-9528-de1375c3e9fb.
26. Eric Lipton, "Food Industry Enlisted Academics in G.M.O. Lobbying War, Emails Show," *New York Times*, September 5, 2015, http://www.ny times.com/2015/09/06/us/food-industry-enlisted-academics-in-gmo -lobbying-war-emails-show.html.
27. George Kimbrell, in conversation with the author, January 2016.
28. Kevin Folta and Lisa Drake, e-mail exchange, October 23, 2014, obtained by U.S. Right to Know, https://www.usrtk.org/wp-content/uploads /2015/09/glad-to-sign-on.pdf.

29. Monsanto Company and nine professors, e-mail exchanges, August 2013, catalogued by *Mother Jones*, https://www.motherjones.com/files/monsanto-sachs-juma.pdf.

30. Kevin Folta, "Anti-GMO Activism and Its Impact on Food Security," Genetic Literacy Project, December 4, 2014, https://geneticliteracyproject.org/2014/12/04/anti-gmo-activism-and-its-impact-on-food-security/.

31. Eric Lipton, "Food Industry Enlisted Academics in G.M.O. Lobbying War, Emails Show," *New York Times*, September 5, 2015, http://www.nytimes.com/2015/09/06/us/food-industry-enlisted-academics-in-gmo-lobbying-war-emails-show.html.

32. Christie Ly (Ketchum for Council for Biotechnology Information) and Kevin Folta, e-mail exchange, May 30, 2013, https://www.documentcloud.org/documents/2303691-kevin-folta-uoffloridadocs.html#document/p84/a237719.

33. Eric Lipton, "Food Industry Enlisted Academics in G.M.O. Lobbying War, Emails Show," *New York Times*, September 5, 2015, http://www.nytimes.com/2015/09/06/us/food-industry-enlisted-academics-in-gmo-lobbying-war-emails-show.html.

34. Emily Schmidt (Ketchum) to Kevin Folta, e-mail, July 31, 2013, obtained by U.S. Right to Know, http://www.gmo.news/kevin-folta-gmo-monsanto-emails-university-of-florida.txt.

35. Kevin Folta, "From This Expert," GMO Answers, July 29, 2013, https://gmoanswers.com/experts/kevin-folta?page=9.

36. *New York Times*, DocumentCloud, 2303691-kevin-folta-uoffloridadocs, p. 104, https://www.documentcloud.org/documents/2303691-kevin-folta-uoffloridadocs.html#document/p84/a237719.

37. Kevin Folta, "Kevin Folta on Winning Borlaug Ag Comm Award, Year of Attacks from Anti-GMO Activists," Genetic Literacy Project, April 21, 2016, https://www.geneticliteracyproject.org/2016/04/21/kevin-folta-reflects-winning-ag-comm-award-year-attacks-anti-gmo-activists/.

38. Council for Agricultural Science and Technology, "Dr. Kevin Folta Chosen as 2016 Borlaug CAST Communication Award Winner," April 25, 2016. For general information about the award, see http://www.cast-science.org/borlaug_cast_communication_award/.

39. Gary Ruskin, in conversation with the author, January 2017.

40. *New York Times*, DocumentCloud, 2303691-kevin-folta-uoffloridadocs, p. 168, https://www.documentcloud.org/documents/2303691-kevin-folta -uoffloridadocs.html#document/p84/a237719.

41. Monsanto Company, e-mails to Kevin Folta, January 2012, catalogued by *Mother Jones*, https://www.motherjones.com/files/webmd.pdf.

42. Anna Lappé, "Big Food Uses Mommy Bloggers to Shape Public Opinion," *Al Jazeera America*, August 1, 2014, http://america.aljazeera.com/opinions /2014/8/food-agriculturemonsantogmoadvertising.html.

43. U.S. District Court for the Northern District of California, In Re: Round-up Products Liability Litigation, Case No. 3:16-md-02741-VC, Document 246-2, filed April 20, 2017, p. 2, https://usrtk.org/wp-content/uploads /2017/04/MDLLetNothingGomotion.pdf.

44. Vani Hari, "The Unethical Tactics of the Chemical Industry to Silence the Truth," *Food Babe* (blog), October 6, 2016, http://foodbabe.com /2016/10/06/the-unethical-tactics-of-the-chemical-industry-to-silence -the-truth/.

45. Vani Hari, in conversation with the author, October 2016.

46. Andy Kroll and Jeremy Schulman, "Leaked Documents Reveal the Secret Finances of a Pro-Industry Science Group," *Mother Jones*, October 28, 2013, http://www.motherjones.com/politics/2013/10/american-council-science -health-leaked-documents-fundraising.

47. Alex Berezow, "Glyphosate: A Slow But Steady Vindication," American Council on Science and Health, September 30, 2016, http://acsh.org/news /2016/09/30/glyphosate-slow-steady-vindication-10239.

48. Alex Berezow, "Glyphosate: NYT's Danny Hakim Is Lying to You," American Council on Science and Health, March 15, 2017, http://www .acsh.org/news/2017/03/15/glyphosate-nyts-danny-hakim-lying-you -11001.

49. Kim McGuire, "Museum of Natural Science Cancels Controversial Scientist's Lecture," *Houston Chronicle*, March 29, 2016, http://www.houston chronicle.com/news/houston-texas/houston/article/Museum-of-Natural -Science-cancels-controversial-7216299.php.

50. American Chemistry Council, Campaign for Accuracy in Public Health Research, January 2017, http://campaignforaccuracyinpublichealthresearch .com/about/.

51. Michele Simon, "Best Public Relations Money Can Buy—A Guide to Food Industry Front Groups," *Huffington Post*, May 16, 2013, http://www.huffing tonpost.com/michele-simon/best-public-relations-mon_b_3273159.html.

52. Nancy L. Swanson, "Glyphosate Re-assessment in Europe Is Corrupt: Toxicology," July 2014, https://www.academia.edu/7595699/Glyphosate _reassessment_in_Europe_is_corrupt_Toxicology.

53. Frederick vom Saal et al., "Response to Glyphosate IARC Attack No, California, Roundup Won't Give You Cancer—LA Times 4-28-17," https://usrtk .org/wp-content/uploads/2017/05/Response-to-Kelly-and-Miller-LA -Times-Glyphosate-4-28-17-FVS-NOTES-bb2-F...-1-3.pdf.

Chapter 7: A Poisoned Paradise

1. Virginia A. Rauh et al., "Brain Anomalies in Children Exposed Prenatally to a Common Organophosphate Pesticide," *Proceedings of the National Academy of Sciences of the United States of America* 109, no. 20 (April 20, 2012): 7871–7876, doi:10.1073/pnas.1203396109.

2. Philippe Grandjean and Philip Landrigan, "Neurobehavioral Effects of Developmental Toxicity," *Lancet Neurology* 13, no. 3 (March 2014): 330–338, doi:10.1016/S1474-4422(13)70278-3.

3. U.S. Environmental Protection Agency, "Chlorpyrifos: Revised Human Health Risk Assessment for Registration Review," November 3, 2016, https: //www.regulations.gov/document?D=EPA-HQ-OPP-2015-0653-0454.

4. State of Hawaii Department of Agriculture, "Summary of Restricted Use Pesticides Sold in 2014," http://hdoa.hawaii.gov/pi/files/2015/04/SUM MARY-ALLSALES-2014.pdf.

5. Bernard Riola, Surachat Chatkupt, Kupono Chong-Hanssen, and Jim Raelson (physicians), letter to Kauai County Council, July 29, 2013, https:// www.stoppoisoningparadise.org/doctors-and-nurses-letters-to-mayor.

6. Qing X. Li, Jun Wang, and Robert Boesch, University of Hawaii Department of Molecular Biosciences and Bioengineering, "Final Project Report for Kauai Air Sampling Study," March 15, 2013, http://hdoa.hawaii.gov/wp -content/uploads/2013/01/Waimea-Canyon-Air-Study.pdf.

7. Paul Koberstein, "The Kauai Cocktail," *Cascadia Times*, June 16, 2014, http: //times.org/2014/06/16/kauai-cocktail/.

8. Lee Evslin, in conversation with the author, October 2016.

9. Peter S. Adler and Keith Mattson, letter to Scott Enright and Bernard P. Carvalho Jr., May 25, 2016, http://www.accord3.com/docs/GM-Pesticides/report/JFF%20Kauai%20Transmittal%20Letter.pdf.

10. Adam Asquith et al., "Pesticide Use By Large Agribusinesses on Kaua'i: Findings and Recommendations of the Joint Fact Finding Study Group," May 25, 2016, https://jffkauai.files.wordpress.com/2015/10/jff-kauai-final-report1.pdf.

11. Pat Gegen et al., petition letter to Libby Vianu and Robert Knowles (Centers for Disease Control and Prevention, Agency for Toxic Substances and Disease Registry, Region 9), October 10, 2014, https://goo.gl/ofRBmE.

12. Ileana Arias (director, Division of Community Health Investigations, Agency for Toxic Substances and Disease Registry), letter to Pat Gegen, August 15, 2016, https://goo.gl/rR9aoZ.

13. "Monsanto Sues Hawaii County over GMO Ban," RT, November 14, 2014, https://www.rt.com/usa/205655-monsanto-dow-gmo-hawaii/.

14. Andrew Pollack, "Unease in Hawaii's Cornfields," *New York Times*, October 7, 2013, http://www.nytimes.com/2013/10/08/business/fight-over-genetically-altered-crops-flares-in-hawaii.html?_r=1.

15. Hawaii State Department of Health and Hawaii Department of Agriculture, "2013–14 State Wide Pesticide Sampling Pilot Project: Presentation of Preliminary Findings to the 2014 2nd Annual Joint Government Water Quality Conference, Wailuki, Maui, August 12, 2014," http://health.hawaii.gov/sdwb/files/2014/09/03.Maui-WQP-Pesticide-Presentation.pdf.

16. "Pesticide Ban to Be Considered in Hawaii County," Big Island Video News, July 31, 2015, http://www.bigislandvideonews.com/2015/07/31/pesticide-ban-to-be-considered-in-hawaii-county/.

17. Keoki Kerr, "Pro-GMO Companies Spend $8 Million to Fight Maui Initiative," *Hawaii News Now*, October 28, 2014.

18. Gary Hooser, in conversation with the author, October 2016.

19. Ibid.

20. Paul Achitoff, in conversation with the author, November 2016.

21. Sadie Costello et al., "Parkinson's Disease and Residential Exposure to Maneb and Paraquat from Agricultural Applications in the Central Valley of California," *American Journal of Epidemiology* 169, no. 8 (April 15, 2009): 919–926, doi:10.1093/aje/kwp006.

22. Paul Achitoff (Earthjustice), letter to Gina McCarthy (EPA administrator), August 4, 2016, https://drive.google.com/file/d/0B-pJR4cGo9ckVVZ2c E9WMlVKZEk/view?usp=sharing.

23. Paul Achitoff (Earthjustice), letter to Lilian Dorka (EPA acting director, Office of Civil Rights) and Daria Neal (U.S. Department of Justice deputy chief, Civil Rights Division), September 14, 2016, https://drive.google.com /file/d/0B-pJR4cGo9ckSi1BT1JTRUZsbU0/view?usp=sharing.

24. Paul Achitoff, in conversation with the author, November 2016.

25. Peter Adler, in conversation with the author, November 2016.

Chapter 8: Angst in Argentina

1. National University of Córdoba, Argentina, Faculty of Medical Sciences, "Report of 1st National Meeting of Physicians of Fumigated Villages," October 22, 2010, http://reduas.com.ar/informe-encuentro-medicos-pueblos -fumigados/.

2. Video interview with Sofia Gatica, 2012 recipient of the Goldman Environmental Prize, South and Central America, http://www.goldmanprize.org /recipient/sofia-gatica/.

3. Lucia Graves, "Sofia Gatica, Argentine Activist, Faced Anonymous Death Threats for Fighting Monsanto Herbicide," *Huffington Post*, May 3, 2012, http://www.huffingtonpost.com/2012/05/03/argentine-activist-sofia -gatica-monsanto_n_1475659.html.

4. National University of Córdoba, Argentina, Faculty of Medical Sciences, "Report of 1st National Meeting of Physicians of Fumigated Villages," October 22, 2010, http://reduas.com.ar/informe-encuentro-medicos-pueblos -fumigados/.

5. Michael Warren and Natacha Pisarenko, "Argentines Link Health Problems to Agrochemicals," Associated Press, October 20, 2013, http://big story.ap.org/article/argentines-link-health-problems-agrochemicals-2.

6. National University of Rosario, Argentina, Faculty of Medical Sciences, "Declaration of 2nd Meeting of Physicians of Sprayed and Fumigated Towns and Villages," July 5, 2011, http://reduas.com.ar/declaration-of-2nd -meeting-of-physicians-of-sprayed-and-fumigated-towns-and-villages/.

7. University of Buenos Aires, Faculty of Medicine, "Declaration of the 3rd National Congress of Physicians of Fumigated Peoples," November 24,

2015, http://reduas.com.ar/declaracion-del-3o-congreso-nacional-de-medi
cos-de-pueblos-fumigados/.

8. Elizabeth Grossman, "A Town Demands Protection from Pesticides," *National Geographic*, February 23, 2016, http://news.nationalgeographic.com/2016/02/160223-photograph-aixa-argentina-avia-terai-pesticides-glyphosate/.

9. Michael Warren and Natacha Pisarenko, "Argentines Link Health Problems to Agrochemicals," Associated Press, October 20, 2013, http://bigstory.ap.org/article/argentines-link-health-problems-agrochemicals-2.

10. Alejandra Paganelli et al., "Glyphosate-Based Herbicides Produce Teratogenic Effects on Vertebrates by Impairing Retinoic Acid Signaling," *Chemical Research in Toxicology* 23, no. 10 (August 9, 2010): 1586–1595, doi:10.1021/tx1001749 (full study can be viewed at http://big.assets.huffingtonpost.com/carrasco_0.pdf).

11. Lucia Graves, "Roundup: Birth Defects Caused by World's Top-Selling Weedkiller, Scientists Say," *Huffington Post*, June 24, 2011, http://www.huffingtonpost.com/2011/06/24/roundup-scientists-birth-defects_n_883578.html.

12. Michael Antoniou et al., "GM Soy: Sustainable? Responsible?" GLS Gemeinschaftsbank eG, September 2010, http://www.gmwatch.org/files/GMsoy_SustainableResponsible_Sept2010.pdf.

13. Monsanto Company, "Argentina and Pesticides," *Beyond the Rows* (blog), http://monsantoblog.com/2013/10/21/argentina-and-pesticides/.

14. Donna Farmer, "Frequently Asked Questions about Glyphosate," GMO Answers, p. 7, https://gmoanswers.com/sites/default/files/glyphosate-and-GMOs_FrequentlyAskedQuestions_Booklet.pdf.

15. Ezequiel Adamovsky, "Andres Carrasco vs Monsanto," teleSUR, October 1, 2014, http://www.telesurtv.net/english/opinion/Andres-Carrasco-vs-Monsanto-20141001-0090.html.

16. "Andres Carrasco Dies; Argentine Neuroscientist Showed Monsanto's Glyphosate Damages Embryos," Associated Press, May 10, 2014, http://www.foxnews.com/world/2014/05/10/andres-carrasco-dies-argentine-neuroscientist-showed-monsanto-glyphosate.html.

17. Javier Souza, in conversation with the author, November 2016.

18. Antonio Emilio Hupan, et al. v. Monsanto Company, et al., Case No. N12C-02-171-VLM in the Superior Court of the State of Delaware, Janu-

ary 29, 2016, http://www.aboutlawsuits.com/wp-content/uploads/2016-1
-29-roundup-birthdefects-complaint.pdf.

19. Antonio Emilio Hupan, et al., v. Alliance One International, Inc., et al.;
Case No. N12C-02-171-VLM in the Superior Court of the State of Delaware in and for New Castle County, November 30, 2015, http://cases.justia
.com/delaware/superior-court/2015-n12c-02-171.pdf?ts=1449162058.

20. "Glyphosate Herbicide, a Catalyst for Argentine Politics," diplomatic cable,
May 7, 2009.

21. Ibid.

22. Connie Veillette and Carolina Navarrette-Frias, "Drug Crop Eradication
and Alternative Development in the Andes," Congressional Research Service
Report RL33163, November 18, 2005, https://file.wikileaks.org/file/crs
/RL33163.pdf.

23. "Glyphosate Takes Another Hit in Ecuador," diplomatic cable, July 9,
2007, https://wikileaks.org/plusd/cables/07QUITO1553_a.html.

24. Pablo Jaramillo Viteri and Chris Kraul, "Colombia to Pay Ecuador
$15 Million to Settle Coca Herbicide Suit," Los Angeles Times, Septem-
ber 16, 2013, http://articles.latimes.com/2013/sep/16/world/la-fg-wn-ecua
dor-colombia-coca-herbicide-lawsuit-20130916.

25. Carey Gillam, "U.S. Tax Dollars Promote Monsanto's GMO Crops Overseas: Report," Reuters, May 14, 2013, http://www.reuters.com/article/us-usa
-gmo-report-idUSBRE94D0IL20130514.

26. Food & Water Watch, "Biotech Ambassadors: How the U.S. State Department Promotes the Seed Industry's Global Agenda," May 2013, http://www
.foodandwaterwatch.org/insight/biotech-ambassadors.

27. Pamm Larry, in conversation with the author, November 2016.

28. Evan Abramson, "Soy: A Hunger for Land," NACLA Report on the Amer-
icas, May 2009, https://nacla.org/soyparaguay.

29. Judy Hatcher, in conversation with the author, November 2016.

Chapter 9: Uproar in Europe

1. European Parliament, "Glyphosate: Authorise for Just Seven Years and Professional Uses Only, Urge MEPs," press release, April 13, 2016, http://www
.europarl.europa.eu/news/en/news-room/20160407IPR21781/glyphosate
-authorise-for-just-seven-years-and-professional-uses-only-urge-meps.

2. United Nations General Assembly, "Report of the United Nations Conference on Environment and Development (Rio de Janeiro, 3–14 June 1992)," August 12, 1992, http://www.un.org/documents/ga/conf151/aconf15126 -1annex1.htm/.

3. Steve Suppan, "Backgrounder on WTO Dispute: U.S. vs. EC Biotech Products Case," Institute for Agriculture and Trade Policy, September 2005, http://www.iatp.org/files/451_2_76644.pdf.

4. "GM Crops 'Won't Solve Hunger,'" CNN, May 28, 2003, http://www.cnn .com/2003/TECH/science/05/28/gmcrops/index.html?_s=PM:TECH.

5. Robin Mesnage et al., "Glyphosate Exposure in a Farmer's Family," *Journal of Environmental Protection* 3 (September 2012): 1001–1003, doi:10.4236 /jep.2012.39115.

6. Jim Manson, "Soil Association Calls for UK Glyphosate Ban," Natural Products News, July 15, 2015, http://www.naturalproductsonline.co.uk/soil -association-calls-for-uk-glyphosate-ban/.

7. Green Party, "Green Party MEPs Peed Off with Glyphosate Test Results," press release, May 13, 2016, https://www.greenparty.org.uk/news /2016/05/13/green-party-meps-peed-off-with-glyphosate-test-results/.

8. Oscar Schneider, "Increased Glyphosate Concentrations in Urine of MEPs," *Brussels Times*, May 13, 2016, http://www.brusselstimes.com/brussels /5600/increased-glyphosate-concentrations-in-urine-of-meps.

9. Nicole Sagener, "Overwhelming Majority of Germans Contaminated by Glyphosate," EURACTIV Network, March 6, 2016, https://www.euractiv .com/section/agriculture-food/news/overwhelming-majority-of-germans -contaminated-by-glyphosate/.

10. Umwelt Bundesamt, "Plant Protection: Less Is Best and Lower-Risk," press release, January 22, 2016, https://www.umweltbundesamt.de/en/press/press information/plant-protection-less-is-best-lower-risk.

11. Nicole Sagener, "Overwhelming Majority of Germans Contaminated by Glyphosate," EURACTIV Network, March 6, 2016, https://www.euractiv .com/section/agriculture-food/news/overwhelming-majority-of-germans -contaminated-by-glyphosate/.

12. Bundesinstitut für Risikobewertung, "Glyphosate in the Urine: Even for Children, the Detected Values Are Within the Expected Range, without Any Adverse Health Effects," press release, April 3, 2016, http://www.bfr.bund

.de/en/press_information/2016/11/glyphosate_in_the_urine__even_for
_children__the_detected_values_are_within_the_expected_range__with
out_any_adverse_health_effects-197173.html.

13. Bundesinstitut für Risikobewertung, "More Transparency on Glyphosate: BfR Supports the Release by EFSA of Raw Scientific Data," September 30, 2016, http://www.bfr.bund.de/cm/349/more-transparency-on-glyphosate -bfr-supports-the-release-by-efsa-of-raw-scientific-data.pdf.

14. European Food Safety Authority, "Conclusion on the Peer Review of the Pesticide Risk Assessment of the Active Substance Glyphosate," *EFSA Journal* 13, no. 11 (2015): 4302, doi:10.2903/j.efsa.2015.4302, https://www.efsa .europa.eu/en/efsajournal/pub/4302.

15. European Food Safety Authority, "Glyphosate: EFSA Updates Toxicological Profile," press release, November 12, 2105, https://www.efsa.europa.eu/en /press/news/151112.

16. Arthur Neslen, "EU Declared Monsanto Weedkiller Safe After Intervention from Controversial US Official," *The Guardian*, May 24, 2017, https://amp .theguardian.com/environment/2017/may/24/eu-declared-monsanto -weedkiller-safe-after-intervention-from-controversial-us-official.

17. Daniel J. Jenkins (Monsanto), e-mail to Tracey L. Reynolds (Monsanto), September 3, 2015, https://drive.google.com/file/d/0B-pJR4cGo9ckSEtrNEE 4OHpwb3c/view.

18. GTF—Glyphosate Task Force website, http://www.glyphosatetaskforce .org/.

19. Greenpeace European Unit, "EU Whitewash on Cancer Risk from World's Most Used Weedkiller," press release, November 12, 2015, http://www.green peace.org/eu-unit/en/News/2015/EU-whitewash-on-cancer-risk-from -worlds-most-used-weedkiller/.

20. Jennifer Sass, "Glyphosate: IARC Got It Right, EFSA Got It from Monsanto," Natural Resources Defense Council Expert Blog, November 30, 2015, https://www.nrdc.org/experts/jennifer-sass/glyphosate-iarc-got-it-right -efsa-got-it-monsanto.

21. Christopher J. Portier et al., letter to Vytenis Andriukaitis (European Commission) titled "Open Letter: Review of the Carcinogenicity of Glyphosate by EFSA and BfR ," November 27, 2015, http://www.zeit.de/wissen/umwelt /2015-11/glyphosat-offener-brief.pdf.

22. Ibid.

23. European Parliament, "EU's Pesticide Risk Assessment System: The Case of Glyphosate," Study for the ENVI Committee, May 24, 2016, http://www.europarl.europa.eu/RegData/etudes/STUD/2016/587309/IPOL_STU(2016)587309_EN.pdf.

24. Monsanto Company, Public Access to Document Team, letter to European Food Safety Authority, February 4, 2016, https://corporateeurope.org/sites/default/files/attachments/efsa_ref._15866348_pad_2016_046_disclosure_enclosure.pdf.

25. European Food Safety Authority, "Glyphosate: EFSA Shares Raw Data from Risk Assessment," press release, December 9, 2016, https://www.efsa.europa.eu/en/press/news/161209.

26. Arthur Neslen, "UN/WHO Panel in Conflict of Interest Row over Glyphosate Cancer Risk," *The Guardian*, May 17, 2016, https://www.theguardian.com/environment/2016/may/17/unwho-panel-in-conflict-of-interest-row-over-glyphosates-cancer-risk.

27. Arthur Neslen, "Vote on Controversial Weedkiller's European License Postponed," *The Guardian*, March 8, 2016, https://www.theguardian.com/environment/2016/mar/08/eu-vote-on-controversial-weedkiller-licence-postponed-glyphosate.

28. ANSES—French Agency for Food, Environmental and Occupational Health & Safety, "ANSES's Opinion on the Carcinogenic Nature of Glyphosate for Humans," press release, December 2, 2016, https://www.anses.fr/en/content/ansess-opinion-carcinogenic-nature-glyphosate-humans.

29. European Chemicals Agency, "Glyphosate Not Classified as a Carcinogen by ECHA," press release, March 15, 2017, https://echa.europa.eu/-/glyphosate-not-classified-as-a-carcinogen-by-echa.

30. Claudia Bolognesi et al., "Genotoxic Activity of Glyphosate and Its Technical Formulation Roundup," *Journal of Agricultural and Food Chemistry* 45, no. 5 (May 19, 1997): 1957–1962, doi:10.1021/jf9606518; published in full on ResearchGate, https://goo.gl/mC6I2l.

31. U.S. District Court for the Northern District of California, In Re: Roundup Products Liability Litigation, Case No. 3:16-md-02741-VC, Document 192-3, filed March 15, 2017, pp. 2–3, https://usrtk.org/wp-content/uploads/2017/03/192series.pdf.

32. U.S. District Court for the Northern District of California, In Re: Round-up Products Liability Litigation, Case No. 3:16-md-02741-VC, Document 192-7, filed March 15, 2017, p. 2, https://usrtk.org/wp-content/uploads /2017/03/192series.pdf.

33. U.S. District Court for the Northern District of California, In Re: Round-up Products Liability Litigation, Case No. 3:16-md-02741-VC, Document 192-1, filed March 15, 2017, pp. 2–3, https://usrtk.org/wp-content/uploads /2017/03/192series.pdf.

34. Philippe Lamberts et al., letter to Jean-Claude Juncker (European Commission) from members of the European Parliament, March 24, 2017, http: //extranet.greens-efa.eu/public/media/file/1/5083.

35. Rolando Manfredini, in conversation with the author, December 2016.

36. Cancer Research UK, Non-Hodgkin Lymphoma Incidence Statistics," http: //www.cancerresearchuk.org/health-professional/cancer-statistics/statistics -by-cancer-type/non-hodgkin-lymphoma/incidence#heading-Nine.

37. Andrea Ferrante, in conversation with the author, December 2016.

Chapter 10: When Weeds Don't Die, But Butterflies Do

1. Bill Johnson, in conversation with the author, December 2016.

2. Roberto A. Ferdman, "The Decline of the Small American Family Farm in One Chart," *Washington Post*, September 16, 2014, https://www.washington post.com/news/wonk/wp/2014/09/16/the-decline-of-the-small-american -family-farm-in-one-chart/?utm_term=.f53170de29bc.

3. Kent Fraser, "Glyphosate Resistant Weeds—Intensifying," Stratus Ag Research, January 25, 2013, http://stratusresearch.com/blog/glyphosate-resis tant-weeds-intensifying.

4. Dallas Peterson, in conversation with the author, January 2017.

5. I. Heap, "International Survey of Herbicide Resistant Weeds: Weeds Resistant to EPSP Synthase Inhibitors (G/9) by Species and Country," accessed December 23, 2016, http://weedscience.org/Summary/MOA.aspx?MOAID =12.

6. Andre Gallant, "Pigweed in the Cotton: A 'Superweed' Invades Georgia," *Modern Farmer*, July 18, 2013, http://modernfarmer.com/2013/07/super weeds-2/.

7. Dean Campbell, in conversation with the author, December 2016.

8. Mike Owen and Chris Boerboom, "National Glyphosate Stewardship Forum," November 17, 2004, http://www.weeds.iastate.edu/weednews/2006/NGSF%20final%20report.pdf.

9. Chris Boerboom, "National Glyphosate Stewardship Forum II: A Call to Action," March 21, 2007, http://www.weeds.iastate.edu/mgmt/2007/NGSFII_final.pdf.

10. Bryan Young, in conversation with the author, December 2016.

11. Patricia Callahan, "EPA Tosses Aside Safety Data, Says Dow Pesticide for GMOs Won't Harm People," *Chicago Tribune*, December 8, 2015, http://www.chicagotribune.com/news/watchdog/ct-gmo-crops-pesticide-resistance-met-20151203-story.html.

12. Center for Biological Diversity, "EPA Approves Use of Dangerous Herbicide Dicamba on GE Crops," press release, November 9, 2016, http://www.biologicaldiversity.org/news/press_releases/2016/pesticides-11-09-2016.html.

13. Chris Clayton, "Farmer Allegedly Killed Over Dicamba," DTN, October 28, 2016, https://www.dtnpf.com/agriculture/web/ag/news/article/2016/10/28/confrontation-herbicide-drift-leads.

14. Center for Food Safety, "Public Interest Groups, Farmers File Lawsuit Challenging Monsanto's Toxic Pesticides," press release, January 23, 2017, http://www.centerforfoodsafety.org/press-releases/4744/public-interest-groups-farmers-file-lawsuit-challenging-monsantos-toxic-pesticides.

15. Stanley Culpepper, in conversation with the author, January 2017.

16. Bryan Young, in conversation with the author, December 2016.

17. Eric Lipton, "Food Industry Enlisted Academics in G.M.O. Lobbying War, Emails Show," *New York Times*, September 5, 2015, http://www.nytimes.com/2015/09/06/us/food-industry-enlisted-academics-in-gmo-lobbying-war-emails-show.html.

18. E-mail communications and other documents obtained by U.S. Right to Know and the *New York Times*, https://assets.documentcloud.org/documents/2303692/david-shaw-missstateuniverdocs.pdf.

19. Ibid.

20. Monsanto Company, "USDA Deregulates Monsanto's Next-Generation Weed Control Trait Technology," press release, January 15, 2015, http://news.monsanto.com/press-release/usda-deregulates-monsantos-next-generation-weed-control-trait-technology.

21. Dean Campbell, in conversation with the author, December 2016.
22. Brice X. Semmens et al., "Quasi-Extinction Risk and Population Targets for the Eastern, Migratory Population of Monarch Butterflies," *Scientific Reports* 6, no. 23265 (March 21, 2016), doi:10.1038/srep23265.
23. Center for Biological Diversity et al., "Before the Secretary of the Interior: Petition to Protect the Monarch Butterfly (*Danaus plexippus plexippus*) under the Endangered Species Act," August 26, 2014, http://www.biologicaldiversity.org/species/invertebrates/pdfs/Monarch_ESA_Petition.pdf.
24. Darryl Fears, "The Monarch Massacre: Nearly a Billion Butterflies Have Vanished," *Washington Post*, February 9, 2015, https://www.washingtonpost.com/news/energy-environment/wp/2015/02/09/the-monarch-massacre-nearly-a-billion-butterflies-have-vanished/?tid=a_inl&utm_term=.1f5b58f87bdc.
25. Pollinator Health Task Force, "National Strategy to Promote the Health of Honey Bees and Other Pollinators," May 19, 2015, https://obamawhitehouse.archives.gov/sites/default/files/microsites/ostp/Pollinator%20Health%20Strategy%202015.pdf.
26. Monsanto Company, "The Monarch Butterfly," *Beyond the Rows* (blog), February 2, 2014, http://monsantoblog.com/2014/02/24/the-monarch-butterfly/.
27. Robert Kremer, in conversations with the author, March 2010 and January 2016.
28. Monsanto Company, "The Science of Roundup Ready Technology, Glyphosate, and Micronutrients: Part 3—Glyphosate and Soil Microbes," September 2011, http://www.monsanto.com/products/documents/glyphosate-background-materials/rrplus%20iii%20-%20glyphosate%20and%20soil%20microbes%20-%20final-9-30-11.pdf.
29. Stephen O. Duke et al., "Glyphosate Effects on Plant Mineral Nutrition, Crop Rhizosphere Microbiota, and Plant Disease in Glyphosate-Resistant Crops," *Journal of Agricultural and Food Chemistry* 60, no. 42 (October 24, 2012): 10375–10397, doi:10.1021/jf302436u.
30. Jefferson Dodge, "Expert: GMOs to Blame for Problems in Plants, Animals," *Boulder Weekly*, August 11, 2011, http://www.boulderweekly.com/news/expert-gmos-to-blame-for-problems-in-plants-animals/.
31. U.S. Department of Agriculture, Foreign Agricultural Service, "Citrus: World Markets and Trade," January 2017, https://apps.fas.usda.gov/psdonline

/circulars/citrus.pdf; U.S. Department of Agriculture, National Agricultural Statistics Service, "Citrus Fruits: Final Estimates, 2003–2007," Statistical Bulletin 1009, December 2008, http://usda.mannlib.cornell.edu /usda/nass/SB997/sb1009.pdf.

32. G. S. Johal and D. M. Huber, "Glyphosate Effects on Diseases of Plants," *European Journal of Agronomy* 31, no. 3 (October 2009): 144–152, doi:10 .1016/j.eja.2009.04.004.

33. Frank Dean, in conversation with the author, July 2016.

34. Craig Ramsey, in conversation with the author, January 2017.

35. Stephanie Strom, "Misgivings about How a Weed Killer Affects the Soil," *New York Times*, September 19, 2013, http://www.nytimes.com/2013 /09/20/business/misgivings-about-how-a-weed-killer-affects-the-soil.html.

Chapter 11: Under the Influence

1. Ted Lieu, "Rep. Lieu Statement on New Glyphosate Safety Concerns," press release, March 15, 2017, https://lieu.house.gov/media-center/press-releases /rep-lieu-statement-new-glyphosate-safety-concerns.

2. Frank Pallone Jr. et al., letter to Greg Walden (chairman, U.S. House Committee on Energy and Commerce), April 3, 2017, https://drive.google.com /file/d/0B-pJR4cGo9ckdmJLdTJuN2pYTmM/view.

3. U.S. Environmental Protection Agency, Office of Inspector General, memorandum from Jeffrey Harris to Jim Jones, March 25, 2016, https://www.epa .gov/sites/production/files/2016-03/documents/newstarts_03-25-16 _herbicidetolerancemanagement.pdf.

4. Lyndsey Layton, "New FDA Deputy to Lead Food-Safety Mandate," *Washington Post*, January 14, 2010, http://www.washingtonpost.com/wp-dyn /content/article/2010/01/13/AR2010011304402.html.

5. Ramon Seidler, in conversation with the author, February 2017.

6. Lisa P. Jackson (EPA), memorandum titled "Opening Memo to EPA Employees," January 23, 2009, http://web.archive.org/web/20100313093014 /http:/blog.epa.gov/administrator/2009/01/26/opening-memo-to-epa -employees.

7. U.S. Government Accountability Office, "Chemical Assessments: Low Productivity and New Interagency Review Process Limit the Usefulness and Credibility of EPA's Integrated Risk Information System," Report to the Chairman, Committee on Environment and Public Works, U.S. Sen-

ate, GAO-08-440, March 2008, http://www.gao.gov/assets/280/273184
.pdf.

8. U.S. Environmental Protection Agency, Integrated Risk Information System,
"Glyphosate; CASRN 1071-83-6," Chemical Assessment Summary, January 31, 1987, https://cfpub.epa.gov/ncea/iris/iris_documents/documents
/subst/0057_summary.pdf.

9. Union of Concerned Scientists, Scientific Integrity Program, "Interference
at the EPA: Science and Politics at the U.S. Environmental Protection
Agency," April 2008, http://www.ucsusa.org/sites/default/files/legacy/assets
/documents/scientific_integrity/interference-at-the-epa.pdf.

10. Ibid.

11. "Congressional Testimony of EPA's Dr. David Lewis," transcript of hearing
by the Committee on Resources, Subcommittee on Energy and Minerals,
U.S. House of Representatives, February 4, 2004, http://deadlydeceit.com
/CongressionalTestimony-DavidLewis.html.

12. Jeff Ruch, in conversation with the author, January 2017.

13. Jonathan Lundgren, in conversation with the author, January 2017.

14. Michael Goodis (EPA), e-mail to Richard Keigwin et al., March 23, 2015,
obtained from the EPA by U.S. Right to Know, https://drive.google.com
/file/d/0B-pJR4cGo9ckVjhZVFhiWXNxNG8/view.

15. Monsanto Company, "Talking Points on the IARC Assessment of Glyphosate Published Online in *Lancet Oncology*, March 20, 2015," obtained from
the EPA by U.S. Right to Know, https://usrtk.org/wp-content/uploads
/2016/09/Talking-Points-page-1-Pub.pdf.

16. Marion Copley (former scientist, EPA), letter to Jess Rowland (EPA),
March 4, 2013, Case 3:16-md-02741-VC in the U.S. District Court for the
Northern District of California, Document 141-1, filed February 10, 2017,
https://drive.google.com/file/d/0B-pJR4cGo9ckUU1OQjJjcVQ4aUU
/view.

17. Evaggelos Vallianatos, in conversation with the author, January 2017.

18. U.S. Environmental Protection Agency, "EPA's Budget and Spending,"
https://www.epa.gov/planandbudget/budget.

19. U.S. Government Accountability Office, "Pesticides: EPA Should Take
Steps to Improve Its Oversight of Conditional Registrations," GAO-13-145, August 8, 2013, http://www.gao.gov/products/GAO-13-145.

20. Natural Resources Defense Council, "NRDC Report: More Than 10,000 Pesticides Approved by Flawed EPA Process," press release, March 27, 2013, https://www.nrdc.org/media/2013/130327.

21. Associated Press, "US Officials Found to Be Using Secret Government Email Accounts," *The Guardian*, June 4, 2013, https://www.theguardian.com/world/2013/jun/04/us-officials-secret-email-accounts.

22. Patricia Callahan, "EPA Tosses Aside Safety Data, Says Dow Pesticide for GMOs Won't Harm People," *Chicago Tribune*, December 8, 2015, http://www.chicagotribune.com/news/watchdog/ct-gmo-crops-pesticide-resistance-met-20151203-story.html.

23. Center for Responsive Politics, "CropLife America: Lobbying Totals, 1998–2016," https://www.opensecrets.org/orgs/lobby.php?id=D000025187.

24. Center for Responsive Politics, "Agribusiness: Sector Profile, 2016: Annual Lobbying on Agribusiness," https://www.opensecrets.org/lobby/indus.php?id=A&year=2016.

25. Center for Responsive Politics, "Agribusiness Sector: PAC Contributions to Federal Candidates, 2016," https://www.opensecrets.org/pacs/sector.php?txt=A01&cycle=2016.

26. Janet E. Collins (CropLife America), letter to Steven Knott (EPA), October 4, 2016, http://191hmt1pr08amfq62276etw2.wpengine.netdna-cdn.com/wp-content/uploads/2016/01/CLA-Comments-FIFRA-SAP-Glyphosate-section-7-10-04-16.pdf.

27. Charlie Tebbutt, in conversation with the author, January 2017.

28. U.S. Environmental Protection Agency, "EPA Administrator Pruitt Denies Petition to Ban Widely Used Pesticide," press release, March 29, 2017, https://www.epa.gov/newsreleases/epa-administrator-pruitt-denies-petition-ban-widely-used-pesticide-0.

29. Megan R. Wilson, "Corporate Donors to Trump Inaugural Revealed," The Hill, February 2, 2017, http://thehill.com/business-a-lobbying/business-a-lobbying/317591-corporate-donors-to-trump-inaugural-revealed.

30. Matthew Herper, "Keep Politics Out of Science, Says Departing FDA Chief," *Forbes*, January 23, 2017, http://www.forbes.com/sites/matthewherper/2017/01/23/keep-politics-out-of-science-says-departing-fda-chief/#58aa046b5f90.

31. Paul Winchester, in conversation with the author, April 2017.

Chapter 12: Seeking Solutions

1. Stephen Ellis, in conversation with the author, January 2017.

2. Charlie Tebbutt, in conversation with the author, January 2017.

3. BCC Research, "Global Market for Pesticides to Reach $65.3 Billion in 2017," press release, November 8, 2012, http://www.bccresearch.com/press room/chm/global-market-pesticides-reach-%2465.3-billion-2017.

4. Sara Mostafalou and Mohammad Abdollahi, "Pesticides and Human Chronic Diseases: Evidences, Mechanisms, and Perspectives," *Toxicology and Applied Pharmacology* 268, no. 2 (April 15, 2013): 157–177, doi:10.1016/j .taap.2013.01.025.

5. Maryse F. Bouchard et al., "Attention-Deficit/Hyperactivity Disorder and Urinary Metabolites of Organophosphate Pesticides," *Pediatrics* 125, no. 6 (June 2010): e1270–e1277, doi:10.1542/peds.2009-3058.

6. Monsanto Company, "Monsanto CTO Robb Fraley Defines New Growth Layers for Company's R&D Pipeline," press release, May 23, 2012, http: //news.monsanto.com/press-release/monsanto-cto-robb-fraley-defines -new-growth-layers-companys-rd-pipeline.

7. Jim Jones, in conversation with the author, April 2015.

8. John Leahy et al., "Biopesticide Oversight and Registration at the U.S. Environmental Protection Agency," chap. 1 in *Biopesticides: State of the Art and Future Opportunities*, ed. Aaron Gross et al., ACS Symposium Series 1172 (Washington, DC: American Chemical Society, 2015), doi: 10.1021/bk-2014-1172.ch001, https://www.epa.gov/sites/production/files /2015-08/documents/biopesticide-oversight-chapter_0.pdf.

9. Matthew Wallenstein, in conversation with the author, February 2017.

10. Organic Trade Association, "Robust Organic Sector Stays on Upward Climb, Posts New Records in U.S. Sales," press release, May 24, 2017, https: //www.ota.com/news/press-releases/19681.

11. Mark Schonbeck, Diana Jerkins, and Joanna Ory, "Taking Stock: Analyzing and Reporting Organic Research Investments, 2002–2014," Organic Farm- ing Research Foundation, August 2016, http://ofrf.org/sites/ofrf.org/files /staff/ExecutiveSummary_V4.11_Web.pdf.

12. Rodale Institute, "The Farming Systems Trial: Celebrating 30 Years," http: //rodaleinstitute.org/assets/FSTbooklet.pdf.

13. Nafeez Ahmed, "UN: Only Small Farmers and Agroecology Can Feed the World," Permaculture Research Institute, September 26, 2014, http://

permaculturenews.org/2014/09/26/un-small-farmers-agroecology-can-feed-world/.

14. National Corn Growers Association, "U.S. Corn Ending Stocks, 1936–2016," http://www.worldofcorn.com/#us-corn-ending-stocks.

15. Greg Stegner, in conversation with the author, February 2017.

16. U.S. Government Accountability Office, "Food Safety: FDA and USDA Should Strengthen Pesticide Residue Monitoring Programs and Further Disclose Monitoring Limitations; Recommendations for Executive Action," GAO-15-38, published October 7, 2014, publicly released November 6, 2014, http://www.gao.gov/products/GAO-15-38.

17. Jonathan Lundgren, in conversation with the author, January 2017.

Epilogue

1. Teri McCall, in conversations with the author, March 2016, March and April 2017.

2. Paul McCall, "Artistic Eulogy for Dad," December 2015.

About the Author

Carey Gillam is a veteran journalist with more than twenty-five years' experience covering corporate America, including stints covering some of the country's biggest banks and the long-troubled U.S. health-care system. In 1998, Gillam's work turned from finance to food as she took on in-depth coverage of the agricultural industry as a senior U.S. correspondent for the global newswire Reuters. Her research has taken her on travels throughout America's farm country. She has spent countless hours driving dusty rural roads, meeting with row crop farmers, cattle ranchers, hog and poultry producers, and vegetable and orchard operators from the Dakotas to Texas and from California to Florida. She has also visited the high-tech laboratories and greenhouses and corporate offices of some of the largest U.S. agribusinesses and met many times with key U.S. regulators, lawmakers, and scientists. Gillam's work has won several awards over the years, and she has been recognized as one of the top journalists in the country covering food and agriculture.

Gillam left Reuters in late 2015 to become research director for the nonprofit consumer group U.S. Right to Know, whose mission is to educate and inform consumers about the often-hidden practices and policies that shape the food system.

She resides in Overland Park, Kansas, with her husband and three children.

Index

Abraxis, LLC, 56
Academics Review (web site), 121–22, 124
Acceptable daily intake (ADI), 59–60
Achitoff, Paul, 148–51, 199–200
Achterberg, Franziska, 178
Adler, Peter, 151
Agent Orange, 26, 197, 228
Agricultural Health Study (AHS), 90–91, 94
Agriculture
    biotech, 2, 44, 48
    chemically based, 237
    decline in family farms, 191
    microbial solutions vs. synthetic chemicals,
        239–42
    organic, 242–43
    sustainable, 243–45
Agrigenetics, 142
AGRO, 209
Agrochemical industry
    campaigns against, 145–46
    corporate interests vs. public safety, 2–3
    failures in oversight of, 218
    front organizations funded by, 132
    on Hawaiian Islands, 135–39
    influence and reach in suppression of
        scientific findings, 5, 181–82
    influence over American academics, 128
    power over regulators and lawmakers, 218,
        231–32
    safety testing by, 217–18
    threats and vilification directed at activists,
        145
    use of social media and stealth marketing,
        128–32
Agroecology, 243–44

Alliance for Natural Health, 55–56
Almonds, 52
American Academy of Pediatrics, 238
American Chemical Society, 209
American Council on Science and Health
        (ACSH), 131
Aminomethylphosphonic acid (AMPA), 58–59,
        65
Anaplastic large-cell lymphoma (ALCL), 21–22
Andriukaitis, Vytenis, 179
Anniston, Alabama, 19
Anresco Laboratories, 62
Antoniou, Michael, 77
Argentina
    agrochemical use and disease parallels, 159–60
    Doctors of Fumigated Towns, 157–59
    farmers' use of GMO seeds, 153–54
    glyphosate ban, 162
    health problems in soybean-growing areas,
        154, 160
    illness and death of children in Ituzaingó,
        155–57
    lawsuits against Monsanto, 163–64
    Roundup studies, 81
    U.S. government's eagerness to promote and
        sustain use of glyphosate in, 164–65
Arias, Ileana, 143–44
Atrazine, 137, 145, 150
Attention deficit hyperactivity disorder
        (ADHD), 238
Ávila Vázquez, Medardo, 158
Ayrault, Jean-Marc, 117

Baden-Mayer, Alexis, 109
Baldi, Isabelle, 92–93

Barañao, Lino, 162–63
Battaglin, William, 59
Baur, Xaver, 180
Bayer AG, 18, 183–84
Bees, 74–75, 204–6
Begley, Tim, 67
Benbrook, Charles, 51, 61
Bifenthrin, 139
BioCheck, 169–70
Biologicals, 239
Biopesticides, 240–41
Biotech agriculture, 2, 44, 48
Birth defects associated with pesticide exposure,
    81, 138, 154, 160
Blair, Aaron, 93, 100
Blum, Kathy, 109
Borlaug CASTCommunication Award, 127–28
Bowman, Laura, 68
Brazil, 80–81
Breast cancer, 84
Breyer, Charles R., 49
Britain, 27–28, 80–81, 173–74
Buonsante, Vito, 182
Bush, George W., 171–72
Butterflies, 205–6
Byrne, Jay, 121

Califf, Robert, 234
California, 21, 63, 99–100, 117–18, 148–49
Callahan, Patricia, 230
Campbell, Dean, 194–95, 197, 202–3
Canadian Food Inspection Agency (CFIA),
    68–69
Carmichael, Nate and Marcela, 75–76
Carrasco, Andrés, 81, 160–63
Carson, Rachel, 1–2, 235
Cell-cycle dysregulaton, 84
Center for Food Safety, 130–31
Center for Responsive Politics, 231
Centers for Disease Control and Prevention
    (CDC), 142–44
Chamber of Agricultural Health and Fertilizers,
    162
Chamkasem, Narong, 72–73, 75–76
Chassy, Bruce, 120–24
Children
    chlorpyrifos exposure and altered brain
        development, 136
    illness and death of, linked to glyphosate
        exposure, 155–57
    margin of safety designed for protection of,
        61, 102

pesticide exposures and, 61, 64, 70–71, 83
susceptibility to adverse effects of pesticides,
    234, 237–38
Chlorpyrifos, 136–37, 139, 150, 218, 231–34
Chromosomal damage in blood cells, 84
Chronic reference doses, basis for and uses of,
    59–60
Cilag, 23–24
Citrus greening (huanglongbing), 211–13
Clean Water Act violations, Kauai, 150–51
Climate change, 205
Coffee farmers, 13–15
Colombia, 63, 165–66
Columbia Center for Children's Environmental
    Health, 136
Competitive Enterprise Institute, 230
Consumers Union, 59
Cook-Schultz, Kara, 89
Cooper, Danielle, 72
Copley, Marion, 227
Core crops, oversupply of, 245
Corporate Europe Observatory, 180
Council for Biotchnology Information (CBI),
    122
Covey, Shanny, 21
Cox, Darren, 74–75
Craven Laboratories, 37
CropLife America, 105–6, 230–32
CropLife International, 97–98
Cropping practices, traditional, 190–91, 195
Culpepper, Stanley, 200

Dean, Frank, 212–13
Detox Project, 57–58, 62
Diazinon, 91
Dicamba, 198–99, 201–2
Dichlorodiphenyltrichloroethane (DDT), 2,
    19–20, 26, 211
Dioxin contamination, 228–29
Donley, Nathan, 38
Dow companies, 113, 197–98, 202, 218, 230,
    233–34
Drake, Lisa, 129
Duke (dog), 21
Duke, Stephen O., 28, 209
DuPont companies, 113, 137–39, 142, 145
Dykstra, William, 35

Earthjustice, 148–51
Ecuador, 166
Ellis, Stephen, 235–36
El Salvador, 82

Elver, Hilal, 244
Endocrine disruption, 83–84, 117, 137, 218
Endosulfan insecticide, 156–57
Environmental Working Group, 20
Enzyme-linked immunosorbent assay (ELISA), 57
EPA. *See* U.S. Environmental Protection Agency (EPA)
European Union (EU)
    European Chemicals Agency (ECHA), 183–84
    European Commission and proposed glyphosate reauthorization, 117, 183, 186
    European Federation of Biotechnology, 118
    European Food Safety Authority (EFSA), 176–80, 183
    Members of European Parliament (MEPs), 169–70, 172–74, 180, 184, 186
    move by regulators to ban POEA from glyphosate-based herbicides, 87
    opposition to GMOs among nations of, 171–72
    reauthorization of glyphosate considered by, 102–3, 169–71
    WTO order to lift ban on GMO crops, 172
Evslin, Lee, 140–41

Farm Chemicals Magazine, 28
Farmers and agricultural workers
    cancers in, 15–16
    coffee farmers, 13–15
    glyphosate exposure, 236
    glyphosate residues in homes of, 91
    kidney disease epidemic among, 82–83
    lawsuits against Monsanto, 163–64
    losses from added costs and diminished yields, 194
    non-Hodgkin lymphoma risk, 85–86
    pushback against Monsanto on Roundup Ready hard red spring wheat, 51–52, 58
    safety rules for, 12
    use of agrochemical concentrates, 159–60
    use of GMO seeds, 153–54
    See also McCall *entries*
Fatty liver disease, 80–81
FDA. *See* U.S. Food and Drug Administration (FDA)
Federal Environmental Pesticide Control Act (1972), 29
Feldman, Jay, 77
Fernández de Kirchner, Cristina, 155–57
Ferrante, Andrea, 187

Flint, Jerry, 122
Florida, 211
Folta, Kevin, 124–29, 131, 145
Food and Agriculture Organization of the United Nations (FAO), 182
Food and Chemical Toxicology (FCT) journal, 116, 119–20
Food production, need for paradigm shift in, 242, 248
Food Quality Protection Act, 61, 231, 247–48
Forastiere, Francesco, 93, 95–96, 100
Formulated herbicides, 155, 180, 184, 232, 247
Fraley, Robb, 202, 239
France
    Agency for Food, Environmental and Occupational Health & Safety, France (ANSES), 183
    National League Against Cancer (La Ligue nationale contre le cancer), 170
Franz, John, 24–25
Freedom of Information Act (FOIA)
    closeted collaborations revealed, 114
    EPA and, 102–3, 225–26, 229
    FDA and, 74
    use of, 3
Friends of the Earth, 173
Fritschi, Lin, 11

Gatica, Sofia, 155–57
General Mills, lawsuit against, 63
Genetically modified organisms (GMOs)
    bans considered or enacted, 117, 171–72
    glyphosate-tolerant trait in, 2, 193–95
    hard red spring wheat, 51–52
    Monsanto's commercialization of, 10
    public policy debates over introduction of, 1–2
    soybeans, 43–46, 153–57, 161
    U.S. government's promotion of, 167–68, 171–72
    Vrain and, 111
Georgia, 200
Germany
    ban on glyphosate in, 63
    BfR *(Bundesinstitut für Risikobewertung)* (Federal Institute for Risk Assessment), 175–77, 179–80
    BMEL (Federal Ministry of Food and Agriculture), 176
    UBA *(Umwelt Bundesamt)* (Environment Agency), 175
Ghali, George Z., 35

Glyphosate
    aerial spraying of, 155–58, 166, 168
    bans on, considered or enacted, 63, 145–46,
        162
    carcinogenicity: EPA Toxicology Branch Ad
        Hoc Committee investigation, 31–32;
        European Chemicals Agency (ECHA)
        conclusion on, 184; IARC conclusion,
        94–96, 159, 166, 171–72; WHO
        classification of, 10, 28, 62–63
    Carrasco's research on, 160–61
    dangers of Roundup vs., 79–80
    discovery of uses as herbicide, 24–25
    as endocrine disruptor, 117, 218
    environmental problems with use of, 4–5,
        203–4, 212
    evolution of, compared to DDT, 19–20
    excluded from U.S. government testing
        regimes for pesticide residues, 40, 64–68,
        77, 80
    genotoxicity of, 83, 88–89
    patented as chemical chelator, 82
    pervasiveness in water, air, and food, 4–5, 20
    reregistration assessments in U.S. and Europe
        (2015), 98
    research findings and protests over use of,
        4–5, 9–10
    residues: in breast milk samples, 57; in British
        bread products, 173–74; concerns about,
        and push for GMO labeling, 3; EPA's
        flexibility in tolerance levels, 5, 39–40,
        59–61; in farmers' homes, 91; in honey
        and soy sauce, 56; in human urine and
        common foods, 55–56, 173–75; IARC's
        findings, 96; in oats, 72; prevalence of,
        in Hawaii, 145; in soybeans, 65; testing
        by Anresco Laboratories, 62; testing by
        USDA's GIPSA, 66; tolerance levels in EU
        vs. U.S., 86; in urine of pregnant women,
        85; USGS's hunt for, 58–59
    safety claims, 40, 87–88
    "salts" of, 30
    on social media, 128
    toxicology testing urged for commercial
        formulations of, 86–87
    use levels, unprecedented, 2–5, 50–52, 73,
        156, 187
    uses, limited, 99–100, 187
    U.S. government's promotion of, 164–65
Glyphosate-based herbicides (GBH), 84–87,
    183, 197–98, 201–2, 230
Glyphosate-resistant weeds, 49, 154, 189–90,
    192–97, 199–200

Glyphosate Task Force, 133, 178
GMO Answers (web site), 123, 126
GMO Free USA, 56
GMOs. See Genetically modified organisms
    (GMOs)
Goodman, Richard, 118–20
Gore, Andrea, 83
Government Accountability Project, 222
Grandjean, Philippe, 71
Grant, Hugh, 97
Green payments, agricultural sustainability and,
    244–45
Greenpeace, 178
Growcentia, 241–42

Hamm, Phil, 24
Hammond, Bruce, 119
Hansen, Michael, 59
Hard red spring wheat, 58
Hari, Vani, 130–31
Harrington, John, 20–21
Hatcher, Judy, 168
Hawaiian Islands
    agricultural land occupied by agrochemical
        companies, 135
    efforts on main island to restrict seed
        companies, thwarted, 144–45
    escalating chemical use and range of health
        problems, 137–38
    Hawaii County Council bill to ban spraying
        of pesticides on government grounds,
        145–46
    joint fact-finding group to gather data on
        pesticide concerns, 140
    Kauai, 138–44, 150–51
    Maui, 144–45
    state senate hearing on pesticide use, 145
    state's failure to provide regulation of pesticide
        use, 149–51
Hawaii Crop Improvement Association, 145
Hawaii Department of Agriculture, 149–50
Hayes, A. Wallace, 119
Health and Environmental Alliance (HEAL),
    170
Health problems linked to glyphosate
        exposure
    in Argentina, 154, 160
    birth defects, 81, 138
    cancers, 16, 84–86
    chromosomal damage in blood cells, 84
    endocrine disruption, 83–84, 117, 218
    fatty liver disease, 80–81
    genotoxicity, 83, 88–89

hormonal changes, 137–38
illness and death of children, 155–57
kidney disease, 82–83, 120
miscarriages, 137, 154
non-Hodgkin lymphoma (NHL), 8–11,
    13–15, 85–86, 93, 187
research results, 4–5
Health problems linked to pesticide exposure,
    247–48
ADHD (attention deficit hyperactivity
    disorder), 238
ALCL (anaplastic large-cell lymphoma),
    21–22
cancers, 91
children and, 234
endocrine disruption, 137
growing concerns over, 237–38
in Hawaii, 137–38
Parkinson's disease and paraquat, 149
Heinrich Böll Foundation, 174–75
Hemming, Bruce, 56–57
Hensel, Andreas, 175–83
Herbicides
annual costs of, 194
formulated, 155, 180, 184, 232, 247
glyphosate-based (GBH), 84–87, 197–98,
    201–2, 230
preemergent, 27
prescriptive approach to use of, 191
resistance to, 190–93, 197, 199–200
volatility of, 198–99
Heyden, William, 185
Honey, glyphosate residues in, 74
Honeycutt, Zen, 63
Hooser, Gary, 141, 145–48
Hormonal changes in people, 137–38
Houston Museum of Natural Science, 131
Huber, Don, 20

Industrial Bio-Test Laboratories (IBT), 36
Industrialized agriculture vs. agroecology, 244
Infante, Peter, 105–7, 231
Integrated Risk Information System (IRIS),
    220
International Agency for Research on Cancer
    (IARC), WHO
gathering in Lyon, France (2015), 91
glyphosate association with cancer, 16
glyphosate association with non-Hodgkin
    lymphoma, 10–11
glyphosate evaluation and classification as
    probable human carcinogen, 92–96, 159,
    166, 171–72

group formed to tear down credibility of,
    98–99, 132
Monsanto warned by EPA of conclusions,
    96–97
2,4-D classified as possible carcinogen and
    suspected endocrine disruptor, 198
work of, analyzed by BfR, 176–77
International Food Information Council (IFIC),
    71
International trade disruption, 3, 72
Iowa, 210
Italy, 186–87

Jackson, Lisa, 219, 230
Jackson-Gheissari, Amelia, 76
Jayasumana, Channa, 82–83
Jenkins, Cate, 37, 228
Jenkins, Dan, 97, 103, 177, 225–26
Johal, Gurmukh, 212
Johnson, Aaron, 17
Johnson, Bill, 190
Johnson & Johnson Company, 23–24
Joint FAO/WHO Meeting on Pesticide Residues
    (JMPR), 182
Joint Glyphosate Task Force, 133
Jones, Jim, 240
Juma, Calestous, 115
Juncker, Jean-Claude, 184, 186

Kansas State University, 192–93
Kashtock, Michael, 67
Kenya, ban on GMO crops, 117
Ketchum, 125–26
Kidney disease epidemics, 82–83
Kidney tumors in mice, 32
Kimbrell, George, 124
Krautzberter, Maria, 175
Kremer, Robert, 207–10
Kuschner, Marvin, 32–33

Lambert, Jean, 174
Lappé, Anna, 129
Larry, Pamm, 167–68
Laybourne, Vicky and Paul, 109
Leaders Engaged in Advancing Dialogue
    (LEAD), 132
Le Curieux, Frank, 92
Legumes, 191
Levinkas, George, 32–33
Lewis, David, 221–22
Lieu, Ted, 215–16
Liquid chromatography-tandem mass
    spectrometry (LC-MS/MS), 57

Lombard, Margaret, 76
Lu, Chensheng, 70
Lundgren, Jonathan, 224, 248

Malathion, 91
Maneb, 149
Manfredini, Rolando, 186
March Against Myths about Modification group,
    130–31
Martens, Mark, 185–86
Martin, Henry, 23
Martin, Matthew, 93, 104
Maximum residue limit (MRL), 59–60
McCall, Anthony "Jack," 8–9, 21–22, 249–51
McCall, Paul, 22, 250–51
McCall, Teri, 7–9, 11, 249–50
McNeill, Michael, 210–11
Melchett, Peter, 173–74
Methomyl, 137
Microbe Inotech Laboratories, 56
Milkweed, 204
Miller, Philip, 97, 122
Miscarriages, 137, 154
Missouri Department of Agriculture, 198–99
"Mommy bloggers," 128
Moms Across America, 63, 109
Monarch butterflies, 203–6
Monsanto
    agricultural division, 26–27
    antitrust probes, 48
    closeted collaborations/covert connections:
        with Chassy, 120–24; with Folta, 124–29,
        131, 145; with Goodman, 118–20; with
        Juma, 115; panel of scientists formed to
        rebut IARC conclusions, 98–99; with
        Rowland, 101–4, 177, 215, 227; Sachs
        and, 114–15; with Shaw, 201–2
    EPA as ally, 96–97, 225–26
    EPA's criminal investigation of, 228
    founding of, by John F. Queeny, 26
    fraud suspected in dioxin studies by, 36–37
    ghostwriting of research manuscripts, 88
    glyphosate safety claims, 18, 27, 87–89,
        108–9
    glyphosate studies, unpublished, generated or
        commissioned by, 35–36
    glyphosate-tolerant crops and increased use of
        glyphosate, 2, 86, 195–96
    grant money awarded by, 207
    Harrington on behavior of, 20–21
    on impact of glyphosate applications on soil,
        208

    influence on regulators and lawmakers,
        12–13, 31, 45–46, 60–61, 96–97,
        215–16, 225–28
    internal e-mails and documents, 12, 101–2,
        184
    kidney tissue slides reexamination by outside
        pathologists, 32–33
    lawsuit against California environmental
        regulators, 99–100
    lawsuits against, 9, 11–12, 15–16, 47–48,
        163–64, 226–27
    monarch butterflies and, 206
    objections to releasing unpublished studies on
        glyphosate, 181–82
    opposition to Scientific Advisory Panel on
        glyphosate, 104–5
    phosphorus mining by, 27
    profits from Roundup and GMO Roundup
        Ready crops, 46–47
    promotion of pre-harvest weed control
        application for oats, 73
    publicly available research contradicting, 90
    requests to, for reassessment of glyphosate's
        impacts, 20
    response to EPA's decision to test for
        glyphosate residues, 76
    response to health concerns in Argentina,
        160
    Roundup patent expiration and GMO
        introductions, 3–4, 40, 46
    Roundup Ready Xtend system, 198
    Roundup safety claims, 15–17
    scientists targeted by: Blair, 93, 100; Carrasco,
        81, 160–63; Hemming, 56–57; Infante,
        105–7, 231; Kremer, 207–10; Séralini,
        116–18, 120, 122, 172–73
    social media use, 128
    stealth marketing techniques, 129–30
    studies and reports provided to EPA, 39–40
    testing of microbial strains, 239
    toxicology expert for, 185–86
    violation of Foreign Corrupt Practices Act,
        167
Mother Jones magazine, 37
Mothers of Ituzaingó, 156
Müller, Paul Hermann, 19–20
Multiple myeloma, 91

National Cancer Institute, 85–86
National Environmental Policy Act, 50
National Glyphosate Stewardship Forum
    (NGSF), 195–96

Natural Resources Defense Council (NRDC), 229
Nelson, Mark, 43–44, 53
Neonicotinoids, 204
Neurotoxicity, pesticide exposures and, 70–71, 136–37
New York Times, 127
Nixon, Richard, 29
Non-Hodgkin lymphoma (NHL), 8–11, 13–15, 85–86, 93, 187
North Dakota wheat farmers, 51–52, 58
Novozymes, 239

Obama, Barack, 205, 218–19, 222
Office of Inspector General (OIG), 216
Office of Management and Budget, White House (OMB), 219–20
Oncogens, classification of, 32, 34–35
Orange production decline, 211–12
Organic agriculture and products, 242–43
Organic food consumption, 71
Ovarian cancer, 91

Palmer amaranth, 190, 193–94
Paraguay, 168
Paraquat, 137, 149, 197, 235–36
Parkinson's disease, 137, 149
Parry, James, 184–85
Perfluorooctanoic acid (PFOA), 113
Perron, Monique, 107–8
Peru, 166
Pesticide Action Network International (PAN), 84
Pesticides
    DDT persistence, 19–20
    drift damage from, 198–99
    EPA's lack of oversight for mixtures of, 38–39, 69–71
    global market for, 236
    glyphosate excluded from annual testing programs for, 5, 53
    growing concern by consumers, 71–72
    health risks of exposure to, 5, 70–71, 85–86, 238
    regulation of, 29–30, 48, 149–51
    residues in farmers' homes, 91
    risk-versus-reward ratio in use of, 235–36, 248
    in soil and drinking water, 154
    techniques to reduce need for, 243
    testing programs, 40, 71
    tolerance levels, differing, 60

unsound safety data for, 37
USDA and FDA testing for, 64–68
use on Hawaiian Islands, 136–37
U.S. government's promotion of, 164–68
Peterson, Dallas, 193
Phillipson, Mark, 144–45
"Poison in Our Food Supply, The" (Vrain), 131
Poison Spring (Vallianatos), 228
Political appointees heading government agencies, 218
Pollinators, 203–4
Polychlorinated biphenyls (PCBs), 18–19
Polyethoxylated tallow amine (POEA), 12, 27, 87, 116, 183
Portier, Christopher, 95–96
Portier, Kenneth, 108
Powles, Stephen B., 28
Precautionary principle, 170, 247–48
Pruitt, Scott, 232–33
Public Employees for Environmental Responsibility (PEER), 222–24

Quaker Oats Company, lawsuit against, 72
Queeny, John F., 26

Ramsey, Craig, 213
Ransom, Joel, 58
Regulatory system reform, need for, 246
"Renewal Assessment Report" (RAR), 133
Restricted use pesticides (RUPs), 136–37, 140–41
Robin, Lauren, 76
Rodale Institute, 244
Roundup
    dangers of, compared to glyphosate alone, 12
    EPA registration standard issued, 30
    genotoxicity concerns within Monsanto, 184–85
    as herbicide of choice, 27–28
    links to range of health problems in multiple countries, 80–81
    Monsanto's marketing of, 8–9
    recommendations for use of, 13–15
    roll out in 1970s, 26–27
    safety claims, 9, 17
    toxicity of, compared to glyphosate alone, 232
Roundup Ready crops
    glyphosate and, 2, 10
    hard red spring wheat, 51–52, 58
    Monsanto's development of, 28, 40–41
    Monsanto's expansion of, 47

Roundup Ready crops (*cont.*)
    research findings in roots of, 207–8
    soybeans, 43–46
    sugar beets, 50
Roundup Ready Xtend system, 198
Rowland, Jesudoss "Jess," 101–4, 177, 215, 227
Rowlands, Henry, 62
Ruch, Jeff, 222–23
Ruskin, Gary, 128
Russia, response to Séralini's 2012 Endostudy,
    117

Sachs, Eric, 114–15, 121–23
Sack, Chris, 75
Sanjour, William, 29–30
Sass, Jennifer, 178, 229
Scientific independence and integrity, future of,
    5, 181–82, 208–9, 217–25, 234
Seidler, Ramon, 217–18
Séralini, Gilles-Eric, 116–18, 120, 122, 172–73
Shaw, David, 201–2
Sheppard, Christine, 13–15
Sheppard, Lianne, 108
Shurdut, Brad, 122
Simon, Michele, 132
Smidts, Jef, 51
Soil health, 154, 173–74, 207–13, 238, 243
Soteres, John, 201–2
Souza, Javier, 163
Special Help for Agricultural Research and
    Education (SHARE), 126–27
Spinal defects, 81
Sri Lanka, glyphosate studies, 82, 120
"Statement of Concern" (Myers et al.), 86–87
Stauffer Chemical Company, 24, 82
Stegner, Greg, 246
Stevens, John P., 49–50
Sue Bee Honey, glyphosate residues in, 74
Superweeds, 49, 154, 189–90, 192–97,
    199–200
Surfacants, 79–80, 87
Swarthout, John, 123
Syngenta, 137, 139, 142, 144–46

Talen, Billy, 110
Tarabella, Marc, 174
Tarazona, Jose, 177
Taylor, Michael, 216
Tebbutt, Charlie, 232, 236
Texas Grain Storage/West Chemical & Fertilizer,
    47–48
Tillage, deep, 192

Trade secrets, 31, 33, 35, 89, 180
Trump, Donald, 232–34

Union of Concerned Scientists (UCS), 220–21
United Kingdom, 27–28, 80–81, 173–74
United States (U.S.) government
    beneficiaries of programs, 246
    challenges and constraints of scientists, 5,
        181–82, 208–9, 217–25, 234
    lack of data collected by, 148–49
    political appointees as heads of agencies, 218
    revolving door between regulators and
        industry, 216, 218
University of California, Berkeley, 149
U.S. Department of Agriculture (USDA)
    Animal and Plant Health Inspection Service
        (APHIS), 49
    biotech crops, oversight of, 48–51
    glyphosate excluded from testing for pesticide
        residues in food, 5
    glyphosate-tolerant crops green-lighted by,
        216
    Grain Inspection, Packers & Stockyards
        Administration (GIPSA), 66
    lawsuit against, for blocking publication of
        research on neonicotinoids, 224
    mission of, 29
    Natural Resources Conservation Service
        (NRCS), 245
    organic agriculture research grants, 243
    PEER petition to protect scientists of,
        223–24
    Pesticide Data Program (PDP), 65
    predictions for glyphosate and 2,4-D
        herbicide, 197–98
    recommendations for, 246–47
    testing for pesticide residues, 64–68
    on theories that glyphosate damages the soil,
        213
U.S. Department of Justice, 48, 215–16
U.S. Department of State, 164–68, 171–72
U.S. Department of the Interior, 204–5
U.S. Environmental Protection Agency (EPA)
    acquiescence to CropLife's demands, 231
    actions to protect monarch butterflies, 206
    biopesticides, approval system for, 240–41
    biotech crops, oversight of, 48, 218
    Cancer Assessment Review Committee
        (CARC), 100–104
    chlorpyrifos, proposed ban on, 136–37, 231
    creation of (1970), 28–29
    criticism of analysis by, 61–62